FUNDAMENTALS OF CARE OF THE AGING, DISABLED, AND HANDICAPPED

FUNDAMENTALS OF CARE OF THE AGING, DISABLED, AND HANDICAPPED

In the Nursing Home

By

NATHAN HALE PEPPER, L.P.T., J.D., Ed.D.

Consultant in Rehabilitation in Nursing Homes
Guest Lecturer, University of Texas Medical School
Practicing Physical Therapist
Practicing Lawyer
Galveston, Texas

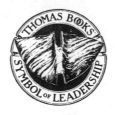

CHARLES C THOMAS • PUBLISHER

Springfield • Illinois • U.S.A.

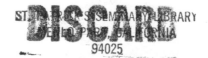

Published and Distributed Throughout the World by

CHARLES C THOMAS • PUBLISHER

2600 South First Street

Springfield, Illinois, 62717, U.S.A.

© *1982 by* CHARLES C THOMAS • PUBLISHER

ISBN 0-398-04637-9

Library of Congress Catalog Card Number: 81-21265

With THOMAS BOOKS *careful attention is given to all details of manufacturing and
design. It is the Publisher's desire to present books that are satisfactory as to their physical
qualities and artistic possibilities and appropriate for their particular use.* THOMAS
BOOKS *will be true to those laws of quality that assure a good name and good will.*

Printed in the United States of America
CU-R-1

Library of Congress Cataloging in Publication Data

Pepper, Nathan Hale.
    Fundamentals of care of the aging, disabled, and
handicapped.

    Bibliography: p.
    Includes index.
    1. Nursing home care. 2. Aged--Rehabilitation.
3. Aged--Institutional care. I. Title. [DNLM: 1. Geri-
atric nursing. 2. Nursing homes. 3. Rehabilitation--
In old age.   WT 27.1 P424f]
RA997.P46   362.1'6   81-21265
ISBN 0-398-04637-9   AACR2

*To the most
important person in my life, my Loving Wife,
Lori R. Pepper
A devoted, patient, and intelligent woman
who is always there.
Without her encouragement, this book
would never have been written.*

PREFACE

THE purpose of this book is to help the staff of a nursing home and allied health personnel to understand all the aspects of taking care of their elderly patients, to give them an insight into their patients' needs and provide them with understanding, and to give them accepted and proven methods of treatment.

The book is divided into two parts. The first deals with nursing homes per se and with understanding the patient in an institutional setting. The second part deals with specific disabilities and the fundamentals of care for their handicaps with total emphasis on rehabilitation compatible with existing disabilities.

A nursing home, through its environment, has an obligation to protect and promote health, safety, and the well-being of its patients. In this type of institution, it is easy to forget that the patient/resident has emotions, intelligence, sensory capacity, memories, self-image, and personalities, all modified by age but still needing and demanding expression and understanding.

Age is a challenge to the individual; it is a constant struggle to carry on life's activities with gradually receding powers. The aged patient has the normal desires to continue to grow, produce, and create, which come into conflict with the frustrations of not being able to do things as easily and quickly as in earlier years.

The reader must realize that the older person's ability to learn at the age of eighty years may be about as good as at the age of twenty years, that society has taught us to be doers, to achieve, not just to live. Understanding aged persons makes it easier to help them achieve their goals. If people deprive the elderly from doing what they are capable of, they make them more dependent on others.

The book has been written in a style that is understandable to all persons. It is aimed to be practical, with diagrams and illustrations, plus specific instructions for the care of the elderly handicapped patient. Each chapter has been organized so that any person can look up a particular chapter that will offer suggestions to the problem that confronts him. Furthermore, at the beginning of each chapter is an outline of its contents, and at the end is reference material. It is designed for people who work to make life a little more pleasant, a little richer for all those who need help — the patient, staff, and family.

A person's fate is in the hands of man alone, but the teacher of the aged person can help him achieve the goals that he has set for himself.

ACKNOWLEDGMENT

First and foremost, I want to thank Ruby Decker, former Director of the Department and School of Physical Therapy at the University of Texas Medical Branch, Galveston, Texas. She has worked hard and diligently on my manuscript and has encouraged me; I owe her a great deal of gratitude for her work.

I am indebted to the Moody Library of the University of Texas Medical Branch, Galveston, Texas, for allowing me to do some of my research there.

I am indebted to Margaret Lucas, English instructor, for her careful study of my manuscript and for the corrections made.

I am indebted to L.T. Gordon, art instructor, for his work on many of my illustrations.

Acknowledgment goes to Linda Carter, who had the hard task of typing, and trying to understand all of my corrections. I am most grateful for her time-consuming work.

Although I have authored this work, I am grateful to all the authorities in the various specialties of rehabilitation for having wittingly and unwittingly helped to shape my thoughts.

Thus, to those people who have written before me and to the many authors I have cited in the various chapters, I wish to express thanks.

I am indebted to my publisher and editor for encouragement to write this book.

CONTENTS

xi

FUNDAMENTALS OF CARE OF THE AGING, DISABLED, AND HANDICAPPED

Chapter 1

THE ELDERLY PATIENT

INTRODUCTION

THE life expectancy for people today is 72.4 years of age. In the United States, there are 214 million people. Those over 65 years of age make up 12.4 percent, and this can be expected to increase. At the present time, there are approximately 1.6 million people in long-term care facilities and 1 million in nursing homes.

The number of persons sixty-five years of age and over in the United States increased from 104 million in 1964 to 185 million in 1966. This increase of 78 percent was twice that of the general population during the same period. The rate of increase for those seventy-five years of age and over was even greater — 111 percent in the same period. These trends have altered the age structure of the population. Since disability increases with age, an increase in numbers of older persons means a disproportionate increase in those who need care.

In the United States, there are 700,000 persons in institutions, and this number has been increasing by an average of 15,000 a year for the past twenty years. There are from two to four times as many disabled older persons living at home, and their numbers have likewise been growing more rapidly than other groups in the population.

THE PATIENT

It is interesting to note that our word for a person who is ill is *patient*. This word stems from the Latin *pati*, meaning to suffer. Our word for the person who is in need is *client*, derived from the Latin *linare*, to lean. It is easy to trace how these words developed their modern meanings, for, indeed, illness does frequently involve suffering and need stemming from some kind of loss and does necessitate the support of another person.

The sick person may try to take advantage of his status as an ill person. Therefore, a delicate balance of roles must be maintained in the world of those institutions offering care for the sick —

3

patients versus those who care for them. The concept of a hospital or their status as human beings. Too often they are called good or bad only according to the degree of their passivity in the face of the nursing home demand for obedience, dependence, and gratitude. The attitudes and care they receive are practiced techniques for removing their initiative as adult human beings and making them patients. They are often less trouble for the staff.

PATIENTS ARE PEOPLE

Patients are not only mentally and physically sick persons but also people who are, or were, engineers, carpenters, plumbers, teachers, artists, housewives, and secretaries. They are graduates of elementary and secondary schools and colleges. They have lived in rural or in urban areas. They are single, married, divorced, or widowed. Like everyone, they all have hopes, aims, and aspirations for the future. Patients have hopes, independence and personal dignity. Independence should be one of the many aims of the treatment plan. Anything done to help in this area has a social, psychological, and physical benefit. All people, including the elderly, are searching for a meaning to life.

THE AGING PROCESS

When is a person called "old?" Some are old at forty years of age; others are young at ninety years of age. Perhaps age is an attitude of mind.

The number of years an individual has lived has increasingly become a way of identifying a person as elderly irrespective of his physical or mental state. It is a means of legitimizing his or her rights to various statutory benefits. Equally important, it is also a signal for employers legitimately to dispose of a person's service and, thus, change the status he occupies in the economy. An elderly person is sometimes defined as an older person who needs help from friends, family, or staff to take care of him.

The World Health Organization classifies age as follows:

Middle Age — 45-59 years   Old — 75-90 years
Elderly — 60-74 years   Very Old — over 90 years

In the United States, some governmental programs classify the elderly as those over fifty-five years of age. However, the prevalent age for the elderly by most standards is considered to be over sixty-five years of age.

The process of aging is continuous and undirectional, which in physical and psychological terms is not identical in any two individuals and varies within the same individual at different times. Aging relates to the changing functional level, whether viewed from a cellular or a complex social system perspective. In a biological organism, it is not necessarily predictable by chronological time.

One of the most important factors in the aging process is the condition of the blood vessels. Hardening of arteries is associated with rapid degenerative changes. The tissues receive from the blood vessels their supply of nutrition, especially oxygen. Associated with rapid old age also is the wearing out of muscular tissues of the bowels and the walls of blood vessels. The replacement of elastic tissue by inelastic fibrous cells is both frequent and widespread in the aging body.

There are four main theories about the causes and controls of the rate of aging:

1. Too many irreplaceable cells are lost, such as those of the brain.
2. Mutations occur in which a dividing cell does not always divide correctly and provide two healthy cells. Enough mutations produce the aged person.
3. The accumulation of unwanted chemicals might produce a general decline in the rate of cell division.
4. Hereditary influences and genetic factors can affect longevity and the processes in dynamic living systems that end in aging and decline.

In aging, the human body has various cells and functions that fail. This inevitable, predictable failure of parts constitutes the aging process.

Age brings with it a great many assets as well as liabilities. Each person of intelligence must train himself in middle age to be ready for the potential later years. We should learn about the uses of medical, psychiatric, and rehabilitative aids that we might one day need. We should not regard aging persons as outcasts but as valuable and essential elements of our society.

It is safe to assume that aging is actually a quality of the mind and the body. The time of onset of old age varies from one person to anothers. As we grow older it can bring a wealth of dividends, including stability and confidence in ourselves, our associates, and our environment. We can discover unique advantages as we grow older; we can learn to face reality with greater wisdom; we can avoid making excuses for our weaknesses; we can forgive the faults of others; and we can try to understand the aging person. Basic needs are common to all people. Each of us needs to feel wanted, needed, and loved; we need to be secure and reasonably healthy.

The potential for the aged to have psychological problems from feelings of being unwanted and of being beyond their prime and usefulness with no future is a tremendous one. If a person has a negative self-perception, he might literally rock himself to death. Perhaps the quickest way to get old is by boredom or lack of stimulation. The simplest way to achieve old age before one's time is the failure to have outside interests after forty years of age. Whatever the real physical or emotional problems of age might be, the person with a vigorous self-concept will endure.

Older persons can have their own scale of values and their own satisfactions, especially if they apply the knowledge and wisdom gained in past years to later ones.

Professor W.I. Thomas of the University of Chicago stressed the importance of the four fundamental wishes of mankind:

1. The wish for security: physical protection and the satisfaction of bodily and social needs.
2. The wish for response: having all the needs of affection, friendship, and family.
3. The wish for recognition: receiving status awards for achievements.
4. The wish for adventure: perceiving tomorrow and its challenges and opportunities in a positive and different way from that of today.

What changes do individuals experience as they grow older? There are two changes to point out in this area:

1. The giving up of social relationships and roles typical of adulthood upon retirement.
2. The acceptance of altered social relationships due to elderly people facing changes related to physiological, anatomical, and health status.

This theory points out that the social and psychologic needs remain the same. The social world withdraws from the aging person, making it more difficult to fulfill his needs. To decrease the aging process, one must be active so that the world does not withdraw. The individual who is able to maintain the activities of the middle years as long as possible will be well adjusted. This individual will find an avocation to subsititute for work and will replace the old friends and loved ones lost by death with new ones. This challenge is present for the patient who enters the nursing home environment, and this is where the staff can help the new patient to make the adjustments to new people, new surroundings, and a new life.

We will discuss the common forms of maladaptive responses that are characteristics of old age. According to Pfeiffer (1977) approximately 15 percent of the elderly population of the United States suffers from significant, or substantial, or at least moderate psychopathological conditions. Stotsky (1970) estimates that between 70 percent and 80 percent of aged nursing home patients suffer from moderately severe or severe mental disorders. Psychopathology is associated with growing older; add poor health, and a double situation is created. Let us look at the adaptive measures that are the principal problems with growing older:

1. Loss of spouse
2. Loss of friends
3. Loss of work
4. Loss of work peers
5. Loss of social roles
6. Loss of income
7. Loss of health
8. Loss of mobility

For these losses, individuals must make adaptations. They should try to replace them by developing —

1. New social relationships;
2. Taking on a new social role;
3. Regaining lost capacities;
4. Developing new conditions.

Pfeiffer points out that there is another adaptive task for older people, that is, retention of function. The areas of function he refers to specifically are as follows

1. Maintenance of physical activity
2. Maintenance of social interaction
3. Maintenance of self-care capacity

Any impairment of these functions in old age may lead to physical and psychological problems. To go one step further for a better understanding of adaptive changes, Pfeiffer points out that there are maladaptive responses that are due to functional disorders and organic brain syndromes.

NEEDS OF THE PATIENT

The average recipient of health care delivery services is a person sixty-five years of age with many basic human needs. These include physical health, social acceptance, a satisfying occupation, recreation, freedom of choice, and a mutual exchange of human affection. Any effective health care delivery system must satisfy these basic needs as well as the emotional needs of aging people. Among these emotional needs are (1) personal aspirations and expectations, (2) self-esteem, (3) self-respect, and (4) independence. Furthermore, social, physical, and mental activities, when limited by diseases or disabilities that restrict these important physiological and psychological needs of aging people, may lead to unsuccessful adaptive aging patterns that eventually provoke mental illnesses.

Overall planning for better health care must identify problems of the aged and sick arising from the normal aging process. Changes in sensory perceptions as a result of this aging process limit the ability to hear, see, taste, smell, adapt to light, and perceive color, which induces personality changes and complicated interpersonal relations. The aging process may also cause physical problems, affecting motivation, vigor, and mobility as a result of neuromuscular changes, muscular weakness, incoordination, adaptive shortening of muscles, immobility of joints, muscle spasms, or spasticity. Defective hearing, poor eyesight, loss of balance or equilibrium, dizziness, or inability to climb stairs even in the absence of disease may further aggravate such problems. Organic disease, superimposed upon the changes of the normal aging process, may further limit the elderly person's activity. The leading organic causes of such limitations of activity, in order of importance, in people sixty-five years of age and older, July, 1965 through June, 1967*, are as follows:

Heart Condition — 21.9 percent
Arthritis and rheumatism — 20.2 percent

---

*National Center for Health Statistics, 1971.

Visual impairment — 9.1 percent

Hypertension without heart involvement — 7.0 percent

Mental and nervous condition — 5.8 percent

Impairment of lower extremities and hips — 5.4 percent

A human being does not exist alone but within an environment composed of living and nonliving elements. All things and people are part of that environment. The continuous interaction between the environmental and human energy systems promotes life. A change in any portion of either system changes the interactions between the systems. At every point in life the human and environmental energy systems are constantly and continuously interacting. Recognition of the individuality of each human being is essential to maximize the potential existing between all energy systems. The following characteristics are listed to help in understanding interactions between individuals.

An individual —

1. is an open energy system;
2. is a thinking, feeling being;
3. has worth;
4. can learn;
5. communicates with vocabulary and mannerisms;
6. possesses learned patterns of coping with various situations;
7. uses coping mechanisms under stress that have previously been satisfactory;
8. has values that are basic to each individual and that
   a. arise from life experiences;
   b. influence one's attitudes about health, illness, play, and death;
   c. affect perception of reality and exercise of judgment.

Behavior —

1. is an expression of wholeness;
2. is meaningful and goal directed;
3. is influenced by how the individual perceives the situation;
4. is controlled by the amount of energy available.

Understanding the needs of the elderly is foremost to treat them adequately as individuals. The needs of the elderly are as follows:

1. A sense of individuality: they want to be recognized as individuals separate from a group or a statistic

2. A sense of belonging to and being wanted by a group: an outlet for social interaction
3. A purpose for existence and hope of achieving goals: if goals are reached, then new ones must be created
4. Provision of necessities: food, clothing, shelter or housing, and medical care at an adequate level
5. Basic material comforts
6. Relief from dangerous debility, anxiety, and tension

Changes that can be noted are the following:

1. Appearance — skin, hair, eyes, and posture.
2. Perception — hearing and vision, taste and smell.
3. Skeletal muscle — Cells make up voluntary muscle; they decrease with age, resulting in loss of muscular strength.
4. Metabolism and drugs — Metabolism is the sum of all chemical reactions that take place in the body. How a drug is handled within the body involves metabolic reactions such as absorption, distribution, destruction, excretion, loss of renal function, and increase in fat.

Aging is a challenge to the individual. It is a constant struggle to carry on life's activities with gradually receding powers. The normal desire to continue to grow, produce, and create comes into conflict with the frustrations of not being able to do things as easily or as quickly as in earlier years. People of a certain age have common characteristics. The elderly may become important because of illness and may use this illness to control their children, family, staff, and the community.

The lengthening span of life takes its toll. It is the gradual loss of the joys of life with the addition of years that alters the delicate balance to which most people have become accustomed.

As their rights and privileges enjoyed in youth fade with the passage of time, biological transition is accompanied either by a spirit of resignation or of resistance. If illness is superimposed or the individual is handicapped by age, there is a social problem. Prolonged illness, sad enough in youth, is sadder in the elderly, if only because it tends to be more extensive and of longer duration when it is entangled with age.

Socially and medically, how can the two be considered; apart or together? Prolonged illness in the late years, when people should be privileged to look back in comfort on a life well spent, is not the ultimate goal.

Everyone should appreciate the interrelation of social, emotional, and pathological forces in the care of the sick. Need for understanding of the elderly person's medical and social needs, coupled with an understanding of human nature, helps in treating the entire person. The type of care the patient needs depends on the individual patient.

PSYCHOLOGIC ASPECTS OF AGING

To deal with people we must understand them. Most people do not want to be thought of as old, nor do they want to be called old. Each must be treated as an individual. For example, a person may be eighty-three years of age, have many physical and mental attributes of a sixty-year old, and not consider himself to be old. On the other hand, there might be a person who is sixty-three years old and acts, feels, and acknowledges he is old. One cannot name a number and say the people who are over a chronological age are old and all others are young. One man said, "Since I am over ninety years of age, I guess I am getting old." So, perhaps this is a criterion — when someone is over ninety years of age one may safely say a person is old.

The psychology of aging is a broad field, including the following among other areas:

1. Sensory and motor processes
2. Perception
3. Drives
4. Motivation
5. Functioning intelligence
6. Emotions
7. Personality development

It is interesting to note that it is difficult to distinguish between biological and psychological aspects of aging. It is safe to say that biological changes do affect an individual's psychological state of being, and psychological and psychosocial changes may affect biological functioning. The authorities in this field try to understand these changes by asserting that the basis of changes is due to instinctive drives. Among these drives are hunger, thirst, shelter, and sex. These experts say that the loss of appetite, reduced sexuality, and declining activity levels among the aged simply reflect that with the passing years drives become less powerful.

Aging is a continuous process from birth to death. Although the rate of change varies at different points in life, all human beings are continuously aging. Growth and development within the individual are constantly influencing the behavioral patterns of expression. Change and aging, in this sense, are synonymous. A change in the efficiency of the behavioral patterns may increase or decrease the individual's capacity to cope with and grow from varying meaningful encounters. Chronologic age represents the passage of calendar time. Biologic age represents the changes in a cell or body structure and function. Biologic age is less predictable than chronological age.

FUNCTIONAL AND STRUCTURAL CHANGES THAT OCCUR IN THE ELDERLY

1. Physical strength: Peaks at twenty-five to thirty years of age, then declines thereafter.
2. Mental potency: Rises to age of forty years, continues more slowly to age of sixty years, then gradually declines to the age of about eighty years. At the age of eighty years, a person's mental capacity is equal to a thirty-five year old if he has had mental stimulation.
3. Physical appearance: Skin — dry and wrinkled, bony parts more pronounced. Hair — grey or white, sparser and coarser.
4. Special senses: Hearing — acute at the age of ten years and thereafter declines. High frequency sound perception is greatly diminished. However, this is not important, as most people speak softly. Deafness is a common problem; this is occasionally a physiological defect, but frequently it is caused by a buildup of wax. Smell and Taste — deteriorates at different rates according to race and heredity. Eyesight — Peak is in childhood, decreases with time. Loss of close focusing ability is due to inelasticity of the lens.
5. Calcium deposits: Calcium is laid down in unusual places in the body, such as the kidney, while in other areas there is a decrease, particularly in the bones.
6. Skeletal system: Cartilage becomes yellowish in color. Discs between vertebra become thinner, resulting in a loss of height of 1/2 inch every twenty years after the age of forty years of age.

Musculature: Progressive weakness and less bulk.

7. Mental age: There is no formula or any hard and fast rule. It depends entirely on the individual. There is some mental deterioration due to isolation, boredom, apathy, lack of stimulation, and the narrowing of blood vessels. The most common mental change is in a person's recent memory. Forgetfulness may come because of deep preoccupation with a problem due to lack of anyone with whom to share the problem. There may be depression and physical fatigue. There is some permanent loss of neurons in the brain. Some elderly will speak loudly due to lack of hearing. There are some functional disorders, and there will be various illnesses. All people become older and undergo changes with the passage of time. These changes take place gradually and end in death.

WHAT GROWING OLDER MEANS

The older person inherits a number of physical and social handicaps. These include loss of physical attractiveness, loss of supporting friends and relatives, loss of status, mandatory retirement age, and lessening of physical health and vigor. Generally, in the Western world, the aged person is viewed mainly as an example of decadence, with no counterbalancing social verneration for his wisdom, judgment, maturity, and spiritual fullness. In ancient and oriental societies, the aged were held in respect. They were the advisors and counselors. Our modern society has drifted to the opposite extreme, where inordinate emphasis is placed on youth.

We must not forget that the misfortunes of age affect the mind as well as the body. There is a greater mental than physical difference among old people. Biological inequality is most fully expressed when one closely examines the intellect. We must realize that the effect of age on behavior depends on the form of behavior under consideration. Significant Supreme Court decisions have been written by justices who are over sixty-five years of age. On the other hand, a swimmer is old after he reaches the age of thirty. The years do far less damage to our mental capacity than we are led to believe. Our minds may have little to do with the number of birthdays we have celebrated. The net result of the aging of the mind will depend a great deal more on how much and how well one has used his mind when he was young. Studies today show that active use of the brain can cause it to grow in agility and power throughout one's lifetime.

Psychological testing does not measure the richness of the human spirit because not all abilities decline at the same rate. For example, verbal abilities resist the effects of age better than performance abilities. There seems to be a physiological basis for the decline. During middle age, the human brain starts to lose significant numbers of cells. This does not indicate, however, that the rate of decline is the same for each person or that every person's intellectual ability actually declines. With the passing years there is some depreciation in the ability to learn, but it is much less than the average person thinks. Motivation plays an important factor in our ability to learn.

Memory reaches its peak in the late teens and early twenties. It declines with age. Its speed has never been measured. The inability to remember recent events seems to be a characteristic sign of old age. Old people remember happenings of their childhood; they forget what happened yesterday. With old age, they become careless of accuracy. Yet, while older people may take longer than younger people to commit to memory a given passage, their recitations are usually more accurate. Although speed is diminished, accuracy is increased.

Age creates few mental problems. It reveals us as we have been throughout our lives. Stubborn or forgetful older people have usually been stubborn and forgetful all their lives. Only about 10 percent of the mental problems in older people can be blamed on age alone. These mental problems could be caused by arteriosclerosis, or hardening of the arteries. Age combined with the previously mentioned diseases shows a loss of fine coordination, easier fatigue, and lack of heavy concentration.

However, we should not consider these difficulties to be diseases; they merely represent a decrease in the efficiency of our skills and talents. The mind has a life of its own, and this mind does not necessarily end its years in atrophy. For many people, old age becomes an exciting time of mental awareness.

We can divide old age into two periods:

1. Senescence: Gradual aging of the body.
2. Senility: Normal aging process complicated by an expected

variety of conditions.

Uncomplicated old age is very rare. As people grow old, their body cells lose their power of repair. Their tissues become fibrous and even calcified.

To maintain good health, all aged people, including the chronically ill aged patient, require nutrition, recreation, medical care, and regular physical activity programs. Regular physical activity provides an emotional outlet for the worries of daily living, enhances the feeling of well-being, reduces free-flowing tensions, inhibits aggression and hostility, and provides kinesthetic stimulation and emotional satisfaction.

REFERENCES

1. *Nursing Home and the Aged Patient,* by Bernard A. Stotsky. Appleton-Century-Crofts, Meredith Corp., Educational Division, 440 Park Ave., New York. 1970.
2. *Long Term Care of the Older People,* by Elaine Brody. Human Science Press, Fifth Ave., New York, 1977.
3. *Development in Aging,* 1969, Report on the Special Committee on Aging, U.S. Senate. Washington, D.C., U.S. Government Printing Office, 297–298, 325–330, 1970.
4. *Aging and the Elderly,* by Harold C. Stede and Charles B. Crow. The Strode Publishers, Huntsville, Alabama, 1970.
5. *Last Home for the Aged,* by Sheldon S. Tobin and Morton A. Lieberman. Jossey-Bass Publishers, San Francisco, California, 1976.
6. *Patients are People,* by Minna Field. Columbia University Press, New York, 1967.
7. *The Physiology and Pathology of Human Aging,* by Ralph Boldman and Morris Rockstein. Academic Press, Inc., New York, 1975.
8. *Psychology of Aging,* by James E. Birren and K. Warner Schole. Prentice-Hall, Inc., New York, 1964.
9. *Handbook of the Psychology of Aging,* by E. Pfeiffer. Van Nostrand-Reinhold Co., New York, 1977.
10. The Adjustment of Aged Persons in Nursing Homes, by B.A. Stotsky and D.L. Greenblatt. *Journal of American Geriatrics Society,* 16:63-77, 1968.
11. *Rorschach Responses in Old Age,* by L.B. Ames, Learned and Walker. Hoeber Harper Co., New York, 1954.
12. Leisure Time Adjustment of the Aged, by L. Calfen. *Journal of Geriatric Psychology,* 88:261-276, 1956.
13. Psychological Aspects of Aging, by Robert Kahn. In *Clinical Geriatrics,* edited by Isadore Rossman. J.B. Lippincott Co., Philadelphia, 1971.
14. Neurologic Aspects of Aging, by Alan Barhan Carter. In *Clinical Geriatrics,* edited by Isadore Rossman. J.B. Lippincott Co., Philadelphia, 1971.

Chapter 2

THE NURSING HOME

INTRODUCTION

THE first impression of the nursing home comes as older persons, with their friends or relatives, enter the building. Is there a reception lobby? Who greets them as they enter? Do they just wander over to the administrative office or other offices? If they go from one office to another, they will react to the atmosphere of the home as they see it reflected in the physical plant, equipment, furnishings, and the attitude of the staff of the home.

There are three basic elements in a nursing home, namely, serenity, friendliness, and efficiency. These elements must be planned by the builders of nursing homes. Reception areas, waiting rooms, and offices should reflect the knowledge that frequent sensitive discussions and sometimes difficult decisions will take place there. The administrative units must be planned to give consideration to the physical handicaps of the elderly. The particular problem is the need to provide offices with sufficient privacy for interviewing purposes, not only to aid the elderly people in communication but also to maintain serenity in a group living situation. Some people with hearing difficulties require others to talk loudly or even to shout. Some older people are frightened and will not talk freely about personal affairs in a strange place or in a place where they feel others might hear them. It is easy to say that they will go to a nursing home, making this decision in another environment, and upon arriving at this home, make a different decision. Elderly people and their families are under a great deal of tension and can be easily disturbed as a result of the visit, due to the environment.

Environment is an important element in the well-being of the patient. There is an interaction between the individual and his environment that is a constant process. The patient through his senses responds to his environment. Doctor Frank H. Krusen says rehabilitation, which is the "restoration of the handicapped to the fullest physical, mental and social usefulness of which they are

16

vironment conducive to this definition. Therefore, it is of vital importance that the nursing home be planned to give the patient the type of environment necessary for restoration.

A person's senses of sight, sound, smell, and touch all cause reactions to the environment. Not only patients respond to the structural elements of a home, but they are profoundly affected by the people who live there. Human emotions interact with their environment. The architecture of the building must relate to the type of people who are going to live there.

In a nursing home, the inhabitants are frequently physically impaired and the environment must be adapted to their limitations. Thus, the space they occupy dominates their lives. The elderly individual's comfort, efficiency, and well-being depend greatly upon the functional qualities of the space provided in the nursing home. The vocational or practical nurse, the nurses' aides, and volunteers are the heart of the nursing home services. These are the people who work all day with the patients. These people must be motivated and dedicated. These are the people who can make it a success or a failure. Furthermore, all members of the staff need to work closely with each other. To obtain greater insight and understanding regarding patients' needs, all members of the staff must feel they are part of a team. Each team member must relate to all others on the team in such a way as to make it possible for an easy exchange of opinions and ideas to give each other access to needed information. To give each other help and advice when needed, it must be a two-way street.

In planning the care of patients in a nursing home, the administration provide high quality health and medical care that not only supplies proper treatment, appropriate illness support, and sensible preventive health measures but also allows for individual idiosyncrasies of ailing people, particulary older ones. Psychosocial and emotional needs of human beings must be considered.

The older person himself constitutes a barrier to good health. Many older people are reluctant to seek medical service. They also try to deny to themselves and others that they are ill. This is a common defense of older people. A patient who denies his illness is trying to conceal his excessive anxiety not only from the physician but also from himself. Such a patient may ignore somatic symptoms and may attempt to minimize their importance or attribute them to a variety of innocent sources. The patient is clearly unprepared to cooperate with the therapeutic or rehabilitative plan or take prescribed medications consistently or for any great length of time. He tends to ignore most medical advice.

Proper management of this condition requires breaking through the patient's defenses to learn what illness really means to him and why the idea of illness arouses such undue anxiety. Is his excessive anxiety based on deeply repressed apprehensions concerning his specific illness? Does he equate being ill with dependency upon others, or consider illness a threat to his self-image? Counseling and reassurance can relieve most such anxieties, but when anxiety appears unduly severe and persistent, additional anti-anxiety support with drugs may be indicated.

Periodic screening health examinations should be available for proper health maintenance and prevention of illness. Most serious disability and illness can be prevented if detected early. Common screening tests are available for the major chronic illnesses of old age. The tests for diabetes, heart disease, glaucoma, tuberculosis, and cancer are easily done.

HISTORY AND PHILOSOPHY OF THE NURSING HOME

The history of the role of the aged and the infirm is most interesting because it is parallel in many cultures. Ancient practices reveals certain concepts that indicate the Hebrew, Babylonian, Egyptian, Greek, Roman, Persian, and Chinese cultures were all involved.

The Hebrews honored their aged parents by giving their maturity a place of authority in their legal, social, and religious structures. They also formalized into law the concept of children taking care of their aged parents. The Chinese, as part of the communes, followed this practice as well. Both of these cultures found that the concept of honoring the aged with the children caring for them in their infirm and aged state gave great unity to the family.

Christ elevated the Hebrew practice to one of love and compassion when he rebuked neglect of parents and commended those who honored them.

The decline of Greek and Roman cultures and the breakdown of civilization brought a period in which the aged were abused, cast aside, and neglected. Following this, religious orders set up way-houses as refuges for the eldery and the indigent.

Then came almshouses. Alms mean gifts. As the poor came to live in houses that depended on others for support, they came to be known as poorhouses.

In the growth of modern nursing homes, the first development was the poor farm. This concept grew up as a result of communities' beginning to feel responsible for their poor and elderly citizens; they would farm out to the highest bidder the responsibility for taking care of these people. Then came hotels and apartments that acted as custodial or domiciliary units for the aged and infirm. Soon the hospitals started taking people in to stay until they died. Physicians would not use the hospitals for surgery and recovery periods because of this association, so the hospitals started to put these people in special sections. Thus, long-term patient care was gradually phased out of the hospital proper into separate wings and eventually into buildings. New names were needed for these areas. They were called many names. Today the hospitals are trying to go back to those days in history and are calling those wings and other parts of their buildings Extended Care Facilities or Convalescent Facilities.

Originally, the hospital supplied the medical needs, and the convalescent facility cared for long-term, chronic needs. Today, the domicile has merged with the medical. As a result, the nursing home or convalescent center is faced with the necessity of providing domiciliary needs and, as its residents become chronically ill, medical needs. The term *medical necessity* is applied to determine the level of care.

Due to government interest in paying for medical services for the aged, handicapped, and infirm people, a definition has been created, which each state interprets as it sees fit. Therefore, there is no constancy in what is called *skilled nursing services*, which is what the government calls *medical care necessity.*

The cycle is complete again. The nursing homes and the hospitals must learn to work together very closely to achieve the medical care needed for all the people who need medical services.

If the nursing home movement is to succeed, it needs to adapt to all types of services. Each must have a definite philosophy. This philosophy must be a working, active concept of the aims, objectives, and ideals of a nursing home, which all can respect and of which all can be proud. Some elements of this philosophy should include the following:

1. The nursing home has a dual role to —
   a. serve as a place of residence;
   b. provide medical care and services necessary for the residents.
2. The nursing home resident will be aged, infirm or convalescing from a medical or surgical disorder.
3. The residents' needs are basically to sustain life, health, spirit, and individuality.
4. The needs transcend race, culture, self-image, religion, or creed.
5. Residents need to reach optimal health and emotional stability through —
   a. medication;
   b. rehabilitation;
   c. personal care;
   d. counseling;
   e. encouragement;
   f. sympathy;
   g. love;
   h. pursuit of independence.

NURSING AND CONVALESCENT HOMES

The needs of older people need to be considered and met in our communities' nursing homes. It seems important to clarify, if possible, what types of facilities are included in this category. Although nursing homes are rapidly becoming familiar sights in every community, there remains considerable confusion regarding their nature, functions, and characteristics.

There are thousands of institutions in the United States offering long-term care for the elderly, infirm, and chronically ill people. These places are operating under many different names, among which are convalescent homes, rest homes, nursing homes, homes for the geriatric, chronic units in general hospitals, sanitariums, health resorts, guest homes, and homes for the aged. Some are privately owned, others are under the ownership of churches, fraternal orders, and non-profit corporations. Some are operated by cities, counties, and other governmental bodies. Some are large, and some are small.

WHAT IS A NURSING HOME?

Let us briefly review the nature of the variously named places. Regardless of the name, many of them are housing essentially the same kind of people. The services they render are misleading, since the names they operate under do not provide a valid basis for distinguishing one type of facility from another. One may ask, "What basis should be used in attempting to classify the various facilities?" Suggestions for the classification of these facilities may be as follows:

1. Their size.

2. The types of buildings in which they operate: Are they converted homes or institutional buildings? Are they part of a hospital setting?

3. Their ownership: Are they privately owned? Are they operated as a nonprofit business by a church, a fraternal order, or other groups? Are they operated by some governmental body?

4. The age of the people accepted for care: Are they only for persons sixty-five years of age or over, or are persons under sixty-five years accepted?

5. The services provided: Nursing service with adequate staff, or no nursing service. Rehabilitative service or custodial care only.

6. The kinds of services needed for the proper care of people housed in a particular home: Residents who are physically and/or mentally ill require some degree of nursing care; others are capable of taking care of themselves.

It should be noted that in too many instances there is a real difference between classifying facilities on the basis of the services that they are providing and the services that they say they are providing. It is important to realize that one should actually visit a home and carefully observe the activities therein to satisfy oneself as to the services actually provided. Two questions to ask are: What is the atmosphere of the facility? What are the feelings and reactions as one goes into some of the rooms and other available areas? The nursing home should be distinguished from other facilities in the community on the basis of what the needs of the residents of the home are and whether these facilities satisfy those needs. Using the preceding criteria, there are nursing homes that fail to provide the basic needs of the people who are their occupants.

An ideal nursing home, as envisioned in this book, is one that satisfies the needs of the people in the facility. In the majority of cases there is a need for nursing care, supervision by a physician, and rehabilitative services with equitable treatment for all patients/residents. It must be recognized that these people have reached a point in life where they no longer are fully able to live independently in the community and no longer have the protection of living with their own families. The nursing home should have adequate services for promoting health, preventing infirmities, and taking care of the chronically ill and the physically and mentally ill. Qualified nursing homes must provide the proper care to the individuals who come to stay in their care.

All the personnel of a nursing home must recognize that the individuals who come to stay at their nursing home have a great emotional adjustment to make. These patients find themselves unable to live at home; thus, they lose the freedom to live their own lives. They must make the difficult emotional adjustment inherent in facing the fact that they are no longer independent, producing members of society and are now gradually becoming helpless to a degree. Residents/patients are surrendering the control over the security of their own lives and destinations and handing it over to the care of strangers. Usually, they do not know how to trust these strangers with their lives. Will these strangers properly care for them? Justifiably, they feel frightened and insecure.

One final criterion for evaluating a nursing home: Is it, indeed, a home? Are the patients treated as residents? Do they have privacy? Are they allowed personal privileges in relation to their rooms? Is it the policy of the facility to make it a home?

A nursing home must be able to meet the needs of the whole person: social, physical, emotional, spiritual, and personal needs. These needs should be determined by the physician, the patient, and the patient's family. The home should have well-kept medical, nursing, and social records available to all personnel who are responsible for the patient's care or who take part in treatment of the patient. These records should be available to the patient's family for consultative purposes.

Today, the majority of nursing homes are proprietary, and economics play an important role in their decisions, whether they are skilled nursing homes or domiciliary facilities. The author feels that all nursing homes would like to give their patients/residents the best care possible. One of the problems of smaller nursing homes is that they cannot compete with larger institutions for the needed health personnel for their patients. Thus, those nursing homes which would honestly like to have a rehabilitative approach in their services are trying to provided in-service training programs for their staff. Not all patients in all nursing homes need all of the professionals associated with a rehabilitation team. The patients' needs should be studied in the light of —

1. the response of the elderly patients to their environment, to the people in the home, and to their general condition;
2. the special needs of these people.

Living in a nursing home for the aged means that a group of nonrelated elderly people live together in the same place according to arrangements planned and administrated by other persons. These homes are designed to give shelter to elderly persons who can no longer live independently in the community and cannot stay in their own homes or in the homes of friends or relatives.

In the past, the nursing homes for the elderly were frequently resistant to change. They have also been slow to understand that the management of their services can no longer remain independent of the community. They are now responding to the changed conditions. This is partly due to the new role of government, federal, state, and local, in supplying funds and services for the elderly people of their communities.

Each person has a different concept of what a nursing home should be, and the nursing home means many things to the people concerned. However, there is one requirement that everyone agrees on, and that is, "The place in which a person lives should be one in which he feels at home." He must sense a feeling of belonging, that the home has meaning to him and to others like him. This feeling of belonging is created not by the building but by the quality of life in the building and the relationships established within it. The type of life that is carried on is enhanced if the building is designed primarily for the needs of its residents. This permits them, the individual residents/patients, to follow a daily pattern of living that meets their needs within the limits of group living; as a result, there is a greater peace of mind for the individual and greater harmony for the group of which he is a part.

A key point to remember is that the elderly patient is a whole person who has desires, needs, and dreams that deserve attention and respect. Life in the home should allow as much gratification of these feelings as possible. The nursing home should make an effort to fit its accommodations and services to the individual rather than to obligate the individual to make one-sided adjustments to the rules and regulations of the nursing home.

It is true that a building itself, no matter how well planned, cannot endow a nursing home with the quality of life that all its occupants want, but it has the potential for promoting that quality by having the proper elements. The element that means the most to the person seeking a nursing home is the privacy of the person's room.

The elderly person who is aware of impaired health, who is worried about the future due to insufficient funds for medical care and nursing service, or who because of the lack of appropriate facilities for care cannot stay at home is looking for a home for security reasons. This person may be alone or may have a family that cannot, and perhaps should not, undertake either the personal or the financial burden of care.

The challenge to the nursing home is to organize accommodations, services, and daily programs of living so that the medical and the nursing care do not dominate the nursing home to such an extent that the home atmosphere disappears. A nursing home is judged by its achievements of proper balance between the demands for care of the feeble, the sick, and the mildly confused elderly patient/resident on one hand and the need for a healthy, normal environment that gives the individual the sense of being at home on the other hand. It is a very difficult task, but it is a fact of life when judging the qualities of a nursing home. The thought that goes into the planning of the recreational areas, lounges, etc., which assures the individual resident maximum independence, should also carry over to those rooms in which individuals must live if they are invalids, or ill, or have handicaps. This will contribute much to the spiritual as well as the physical well-being of the individual and to the entire patient/resident person.

Activities must be provided for all patients/residents, regardless of health status, since many of the activities present in a normal living situation are not found in the nursing home. Privacy for individuals who have visitors and flexibility in arrangements for having visitors are of vital importance. The opportunity for social contacts and religious worship must exist in the nursing home. It also must be kept in mind that if the life in the nursing home is to have the flavor of normalcy, there must be opportunities for engaging in the activities of the community for those who can and wish to do so. Also, it is necessary to bring the community into the nursing home without formality. In many cases, the administrator who has as his goal a home like atmosphere will be able to achieve this goal and bring comfort to his patient/resident.

We have discussed nursing homes that are independent institutions. Now we will consider another type of institution that also serves the needs of the people.

GENERAL EXTENDED CARE INSTITUTIONS

General extended care institutions are extensions of hospitals. They have organized medical staffs that provide total medical services, including services of physicians and continuous nursing services. Their characteristics are as follows:

1. The primary function is to provide treatment for patients who require inpatient care but who are not in an acute phase of illness. They require convalescent or restorative care for a variety of medical conditions. Transfer arrangements are readily available for patients in need of hospital care.
2. The institution maintains inpatient beds.
3. There is a governing authority legally responsible for the conduct of the institution.
4. There is an administrator to whom the governing authority delegates full-time responsiblility for the operation of the institution in accordance with established policy.
5. There is an organized medical staff at the institution, or one that serves the institution through an affiliation, to which the governing authority delegates responsibility for maintaining proper standards of medical care.
6. Each patient is admitted on the medical authority of and is under the supervision of a physician.
7. A current and complete medical record is maintained for each patient.
8. The nursing director is a registered professional nurse, and all nursing service is continuous.
9. Diagnostic x-ray service and clinical laboratory service are

regularly and conveniently available.
10. There is control of the storage and dispensing of narcotics and other medications.
11. Food served to patients meets their nutritional requirements, and special diets are regularly available.

THE AGED IN INSTITUTIONS

It is commonly believed that most institutions have deleterious effects on behavior caused by the dehumanizing and depersonalizing characteristics of institutional environment. Townsend (1962), makes this summary:

> In the institution people live communally with a minimum of privacy, and yet their relationship with each other is slender. Many subsist in a kind of defensive shell of isolation. Their mobility is restricted, and they have little access to general society. The social experiences are limited, and the staff lead a rather separate existence from them. They are oriented toward a system in which they submit to orderly routine, non-creative occupation, and cannot exercise much self-determination. They are deprived of intimate family relationships, and can rarely find substitutes which seem to be more than a pale imitation of those enjoyed by most people in a general community.

In 1970, the number of nursing homes and nursing home beds had increased dramatically. Nursing homes were stimulated by Medicare and Medicaid funds. They grew in size as well as in numbers. Between 1960 and 1970, the number of beds and patients more than tripled, to 1.1 million and 900,000, respectively. During the same ten years, expenditures for care increased from $.5 billion to $2.8 billion and by 1974 had reached $7.5 billion, an increase of 1400 percent.

The result for the individual seems fairly often to be a gradual process of depersonalization. He has too little opportunity to develop the talents he possesses, and they atrophy through disuse. He may become resigned and depressed and may display no interest in the future or in things not immediately personal. He sometimes becomes apathetic, talks little, and lacks initiative. His personal habits and toilet may deteriorate. Occasionally, he seems to withdraw into a private world of fantasy.

Concerning the effects on the elderly after entering institutions, Ames (1954), Learned and Walker (1954), Chalfen (1956), and Lieberman and Larkin (1963) report the following characteristics:

1. Poor adjustment
2. Depression
3. Unhappiness
4. Intellectual ineffectiveness
5. Low energy
6. Negative self-image
7. Feelings of personal insignificance and impotence
8. Feelings of being old
9. Docility
10. Submission
11. Low range of interests
12. Living in the past rather than in the present and future
13. Withdrawal
14. Unresponsiveness to others
15. Increased anxiety
16. Focusing of feelings on dying and death

THE ELDERLY POPULATION IN NURSING HOMES

Most people in nursing homes are old. About 90 percent of them are sixty-five years of age or older. To break the figures down further, 17 percent are sixty-five to seventy-four years old, 40 percent are seventy-five to eighty-four years old, and 43 percent are at least eighty-five. In other words, the greater percentage of people in nursing homes are seventy-five or older. The study that provides these statistics shows also that in the nursing home women over age sixty-five outnumber men by 4.3 percent.

Economically, persons in nursing homes have limited resources. Most of them are carried for a while by Medicare or Medicaid and then rely on welfare. This does not necessarily mean that they have been poor all their lives but that their assets have been depleted by a long period of retirement and inflationary trends. Since women live longer than men, they are generally poorer than men.

Many residents of nursing homes suffer from a combination of chronic physical and mental problems that result in functional disability. These ailments prevent or impair the individual's ability to care for himself in a normal situation. Statistics show the major physical ailments that affect older persons in nursing homes:

1. Circulatory disorders, e.g., heart disease   36%
2. Stroke   11%

3. Speech disorders (usually result of a stroke)   14%
4. Arthritis   33%
5. Digestive disorders   20%
6. Others   42%

Many of these overlap in individuals afflicted with more than one ailment.

As for mental disorders, a national survey conducted in 1972 found that 34 percent of the nursing home population suffered from advanced senility, 27 percent from less serious senility, and another 17 percent from other disorders such as confusion and disorientation.

SELECTION OF A NURSING HOME

The very name nursing home implies that it offers nursing care to people who are sick or require care to some degree. It also implies that it is a resident's/patient's home. Nursing homes, convalescent centers, rehabilitation centers are some of the names of places that come after leaving the hospital and before patients can go to their own homes. Whatever name is given, for many this is the place they will spend the rest of their lives. Therefore, the home atmosphere is more important then the nursing care. There are people who need the nursing care as the paramount consideration, but the same people would like to have the home atmosphere.

The trend at the present time clearly indicates that fewer and fewer nursing homes retain or offer as part of their services the homelike atmosphere. Rather, they are providing the services of a kind of specialized small hospital. Furthermore, they are sacrificing rehabilitative services by delegating them to the nursing staff and not using any specialists in the field of rehabilitation.

The laws of many states and of federal government address themselves solely to extended care facilities and incidentally mention nursing homes as being an outgrowth of extended care legislation. There is a great need for clarification in the care of the nursing home per se.

The United States Public Health Service made the following statement: "Since 1954, skilled nursing homes have increased in number from 7000 to 9700, or 39%. Their total capacity has nearly doubled from 180,000 beds in 1954 to 338,700 in 1961."

A release in the Medicare Newsletter states, "As of January of 1979, 2607 institutions had fully qualified to participate in the Medicare program, representing a total of 188,998 nursing beds."

TYPES OF NURSING HOMES

There are several types of ownership of nursing homes.

1. *Public Home*

A public home is one that concerns all citizens because it is sponsored, and thus paid for by the people's tax dollar. This is the type of home that is owned by the city or county or state and is for the benefit of its citizens that need shelter and care. Previously it was called the poorhouse or poorhome. The public home has now become known as the nursing home or infirmary. Too often it has drifted into becoming an institution without the building, personnel, or program geared to meet the needs of the patients. The community makes the decision on the standards and care given to the patients/residents based upon the availability of funds.

2. *Nonprofit Homes*

Nonprofit homes are voluntary agencies, religious, fraternal, and philanthropic groups on state and national levels that also sponsor nursing homes. It is reported that 41 percent of nonprofit homes for the aged give only general care to their residents. As a result of changes and types of people entering these nonprofit homes, they have found themselves obligated without prior intent to give nursing care to residents because of the demands of the elderly residents who during their stay in the nursing home have become patients. Most nonprofit homes for the aged recognize their responsibility and are giving a high degree of skilled nursing care. They are also making great strides towards improving both their facilities and services.

3. *Proprietary Homes*

Proprietary homes are growing rapidly. In fact, large corporations are forming and establishing nursing homes in many states. These homes are geared to make a profit. They are run efficiently to satisfy the great need for nursing home care. They were for a time under Medicare but soon dropped this because of the higher standards required to be eligible under that program. It is difficult to maintain high standards of care if it costs a great deal of money and more red tape.

The quality of the skilled or less skilled nursing home and its care of its patients has much to do with the health status of patients. The amount and kind of medical supervision and nursing care that are given are important. In most cases, it is important to remember that patients in nursing homes are people whose medical care requirements, so far as direct and continuous supervision by the physician is concerned, are subordinated to their needs of nursing and attendant care.

THE NURSING HOME AND MENTAL PATIENTS

One of the problems that confronts a nursing home that takes mental patients is that many do not have the professional staff to care for these patients, and consequently, there is considerable variation in the quality of care provided. Economy is often a major factor in the operation of this type of facility. There is an ever present conflict between keeping expenses down and providing the good nursing care that inevitably raises costs.

It is true that the State Department of Health or Human Resources is usually responsible for licensing and regulating nursing homes and for setting the standards. Inspectors make periodic visits to evaluate the type of care given and the condition of the physical plant. They try to enforce the standards of individual patient care as well as review the management of medication, treatments, diets, and social and psychological welfare. The Department of Mental Health sometimes becomes involved and tries to cooperate with the Department of Health in checking the standards of care for mental patients. Another department that handles such cases is the Department of Welfare, which determines the legal and financial eligibility of the patient under the law. In most cases, the public welfare case workers visit the home periodically and are well acquainted with the conditions that prevail. Inspectors of the health department are more concerned with physical standards than the nursing care given. They take very little time to inquire about the social and psychological factors that influence the patients. In many cases, if a patient has a psychological problem or disturbs the other patients, then he or she is transferred or moved somewhere else. It is a kind of dumping process whereby patients are taken from nursing home to nursing home. Many owners of homes feel that the presence of a patient who has a mental problem adds unnecessary complication to an already complicated situation. They have to deal with three state agencies, none of which want to take the responsiblitiy of setting standards of care for these patients. In many cases, nursing homes have enough psychological problems with so-called nonmental cases that they do not want to admit an acknowledged mental patient.

That many nursing homes do not have the staff to incorporate recreational activities and full rehabilitation facilities has created a problem that has not been solved except in a few situations. This brings up one of the major problems of nursing homes — the shortage of professional personnel. Many nurses look down on nursing homes and work there only until they find something that suits them better. The morale is low, and there is a high turnover of personnel. There is constant conflict between nursing services that want to carry out rehabilitation practices and administrations that want to provide a profit for the owner. It must be said that in recent years, administrators have been getting better professional training and, consequently, are aware that rehabilitation is part of a nursing home operation. In the past, many nursing homes were built for economy of operation without any consideration of the patients' needs. This has hurt the industry as a whole. Fortunately, in recent years, this has changed, and the environment has improved in the buildings of present nursing homes.

It must be noted that 750,000 patients now live in long-term facilities. Most of these patients/residents will never return to their own homes. There is no federal aid for such patients; however, some of these patients will get help from the Department of Public Welfare. If they are mental patients, the Department of Mental Health will help in some manner. Many of these mental patients are poor risks and have a high mortality rate. Many do not respond well to rehabilitation treatments. They are discriminated against in the present nursing homes because it is neither financially profitable nor very satisfying to care for these patients.

The constant turnover of professional staff leaves these homes weak in personnel. In many cases, the physical plant deteriorates along with the loss of personnel. There is a growing disparity between high cost nursing homes and lower cost nursing homes due to the level of professional nurses, social workers, physicians, dietitians, and rehabilitative specialists who will not work for the lower cost nursing homes; consequently, the latter become primarily custodial facilities. The chronically ill, aged, and handicapped patients require more supervision. As a result of the lack of facilities, they develop more psychological and physical problems. This results in these patients being sent back to the hospital. The hospitals get overcrowded and send them back to nursing homes. This becomes a vicious cycle.

There are signs of improvement, however. Many nursing homes are working together to share professional staff and rehabilitation facilities. The professional staff is on a rotation basis and goes to each home to help the staff in the proper care of the patients.

There is no question of the need for rehabilitation in the area of nursing homes. In the federal statutes on Social Security, a rehabilitation program is actually prescribed as necessary under the "Extended Care Service Program of Medicare." Alas, that is why so many proprietary nursing homes are not part of the Medicare program. They do not want to give the services that are prescribed.

The theory behind Medicare is that patients, no matter what age, should be treated, keeping in mind the goal of their convalescing and being returned to the maximum of physical health, vigor, and activity of which they are capable. Rehabilitation is accepted as a very essential phase of medical and nursing care. For many people, it is the nursing care that is responsible for the degree of restoration to a better state of health or physical functioning.

In a discussion of nursing homes, it seems wise to examine the attitude and policy of the administration and the staff to see if rehabilitation is part of their approach to the task of caring for patients with the goal of improvement of health status firmly and clearly understood by both the patients and staff. It must be said that some proprietors have actually stated in conference that the cost of rehabilitation is one of losing business, since patients will often be able to leave the nursing home for their own home or other places to live. Furthermore, if they do stay, the public agency that might be sponsoring them will have to pay less because they need less help. Actually, one of the newer trends is to have as a goal for the older persons that they improve to the point that they can return to their own homes. This is a realistic goal due to the potential of modern medicine.

To achieve any goal in the field of patient care, one must examine the professional standing of the members of the staff of a nursing home. Do they have the ability to undertake the responsibilities that they have assumed? Are they responsible people in character, principles, and morals? Are they willing to work according to the terms of the job that they are hired for? Do they like and understand people of that age? Do they have compassion? Can they win the confidence of their patients and thus, lead them to improve their health? Are they people with who patients would want to cast their lot, with whom they would want to live if they were in need of tender loving care?

This is what the patient and the patient's family expect. There should be no differentiation between the standards that the nursing home staff set for themselves and what is asked of the patient being placed in the home, who may have little or nothing to say in his own behalf. The needs of the patient should be the primary goal. It is interesting to watch the reactions of patients to those who will be giving them care, for they are quick to sense superficial expressions of interest on the part of staff members. They can detect sincerity or the lack of it with the instinct of children. Persons sensitive to personal and human relationships can be sufficiently accurate in their impressions and estimates of character to be helpful in this phase of decision making.

If a prospective patient and/or his family visit a nursing home, they can get a good impression of the type of care that the patients are receiving by the apathy, general inertia, and lack of interest on the part of the patients. Also, look at the staff that is working. One can sense by the atmosphere of the place the type of nursing home it is.

It is important to think one step further in trying to understand a nursing home. The atmosphere can be felt in the program of care for a human being, that is, for the patient/resident. What is done for them to fill their emotional and deep personal needs is part of the program that is not written down but is done by staff members because they see the need. It makes the concept of the nursing home a reality, which promotes an atmosphere congenial to the person who lives within it.

There is in this nursing home a respect for the possessions of the individual, for the right of privacy, for the right to send out mail and receive it unopened, and the right for them to make decisions for themselves, as long as they are mentally competent and physically able. A good criteria would be, as a patient told me one day, "Where one is treated as a person, not as an object."

REFERENCES

1. A Study of Nursing Home Care. Maryland State, Department of Health, Bureau of Medical Services, Baltimore, Maryland, 1960.
2. Long Term Care Study. Kansas State, Department of Health, Topeka, Kansas, 1964.
3. Needed: Better Care for Mental Patients in Nursing Homes. Panorama-Sanchez Pharmaceuticals, Hanover, New Jersey, 1968.
4. The Situation with Nursing Homes, by O.A. Randall, *American Journal of Nursing, 65*:93, 1965.
5. National Center for Health Statistics, United States Department of Health, Education and Welfare, Series 12 No. 2, 1962.
6. Nursing Home Code, New York City, Department of Hospitals, Part I. Municipal Building, New York City, 1963.
7. *The Last Refuge,* by P. Townsend. Rutledge and Kegan Paul, London, 1962.
8. The Effects of Institutionalization: Attitudes Toward Older People, by J. Tuckman and I. Gorge, *Journal of Abnormal Psychology, 47*:337-344, 1952.
9. Assessing the Quality of Long Term Care, Research Summary Series. U.S. Department of Health, Education and Welfare, Public Health Service National Center for Health Services Research, Publication No. (PH) 78-319, July, 1978.

Chapter 3

THE ADMINISTRATION OF
A NURSING HOME

INTRODUCTION

SKILLED workers in a nursing home must have an understanding and care for their work. In addition to their practical knowledge and education, they must have common sense. If they are armed with these skills and attitudes, the job becomes both easier and more enjoyable.

In a nursing home, it is all too easy to forget that the residents/patients still have feelings, intellect, sensory capacities, memories, self-image, and personalities. All of these are modified by age but still need and demand expression. In many cases, workers take functions away from the elderly. The more that are taken away, the more dependent the elderly become and the more they withdraw into themselves. The loss of a chance to make a decision can be traumatic to an elderly person's self-image. The administration and the staff are concerned with the clinical, preventive, remedial, and social aspects of the health and disability of the residents/patients. The aims of the staff are to restore activity and to maintain independence so that the elderly may live as successfully as possible in the setting called "the nursing home."

THE ADMINISTRATOR

The administrator should have a patient care committee to organize and maintain effective patient care. Its purposes are as follows:

1. To insure that all patients admitted to the facility receive the best possible care
2. To provide a means whereby problems of medical-administrative nature shall be considered by this committee.
3. To establish, execute, and review patient care policies on medical, dental, and nursing service practices in the facility.

4. To provide in-service education and maintain educational standards of the personnel

5. To anticipate future needs and problems.

   Some of the functions to be reviewed by the patient care committee are the following:

1. Admissions
2. Transfer and discharge policies
3. Categories of patients to be accepted or not to be accepted
4. Physician services
5. Nursing services
6. Dietary services
7. Rehabilitative services
8. Pharmaceutical services
9. Diagnostic services
10. Dental services
11. Emergency procedures for critically ill and mentally disturbed patients
12. Podiatric services
13. Social services
14. Patients' activities
15. Clinical records
16. Transfer agreements

Suggested Organizational Chart

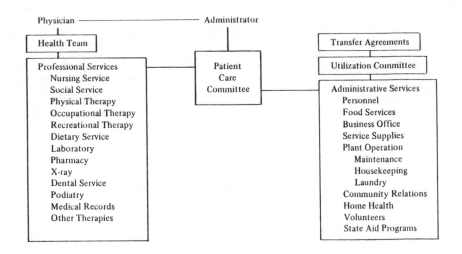

17. Utilization and medical reviews

The administrator must decide on privileges of patients, families, and visitors.

Patients

It is the duty of the facility to provide all the care that is required for the comfort of the patients and necessary for their maximum restoration to good health. The facility must also provide personnel qualified by virtue of their education and training to carry out the responsibilities to which they are assigned. The facility must provide social services to the patients regarding their illness in order that they and their families may best be able to understand and adjust to the illness. The patient and family should be consulted further concerning the availability of intensive care services so that they may cope if such a need should arise. Every effort should be made to make the patient's surroundings as pleasant and cheerful as possible so that the patients will accept their illnesses better.

Families

Families have a right to expect that the total care of patients will be provided in an efficient manner under the authority of a licensed physician and that all rights of patients will be understood, respected, and followed.

The proper authorities should provide continuous information regarding the condition of the patient. A total description of the patient's illness should be fully discussed with the family so that they are able to understand the nature of the patient's illness. This is done so that the family can formulate its own evaluation of the overall care provided to the patient. An official and effective change of condition formula should be available, and the family should be promptly notified when the condition of the patient becomes dangerous.

Families have the right to expect that all health care, restorative and rehabilitative services, will be provided wherever and whenever it is possible, in the best interest of the patient, and that the treatment of all patients will be provided under the written orders of the attending physician.

Official visiting hours should be established, and the proper visitors, including members of the immediate family and others authorized, should be allowed to visit the patient.

No changes in the financial or service structure should be made without reasonable and prior notice to the family.

Visitors

Visiting should be established by policy as to hours and length of visits. Food and snacks brought to patients by visitors are allowed only if approved by the attending physician. No storage of food should be allowed in the nursing unit refrigerator. Alcoholic beverages should never be allowed to be brought by visitors. Smoking should never be allowed in any areas of nursing services, particularly in the patient's room. Patients who smoke may do so only under the immediate supervision and direct authority of the nurse supervising the unit. One of the key posts the administrator has to appoint is the nursing director.

The skilled nursing service is one that must be furnished by and under the direct supervision of a licensed nurse and under the general direction of a physician to assure the safety of the patient and to achieve medically desired results. Nurses have the duty and responsibility to attend to the total needs of the patients. They must plan, organize, and manage the treatment plan as outlined, which, in many cases, involves multiple services where specialized health care knowledge must be applied to attain the desired results.

PREPARING PATIENTS FOR THEIR ROLES IN A NURSING HOME

Prior to Admission

There should be an interview with the patient, if possible; if not, an interview should be conducted with a relative, guardian, or family members. Discuss the nursing home policies on finances, visitors, Medicare and Medicaid requirements, arrangements concerning pharmaceuticals, physician in charge, and house physician in case of emergencies. If the patient is on welfare, his caseworker should participate in the discussion.

Upon Admission

The director of nursing and the administrator should be at the

door to welcome the patients. Be careful to introduce the personnel
who are to work with them. Be sure to assign a licensed vocational
nurse (LVN) or aide to assist the new patients to their rooms. This
nurse or aide should stay with them a reasonable time until the patients seem not to be apprehensive of their new surroundings. As
staff members take the patients into their rooms, they should make a
complete and thorough assessment of the room. They show them the
bathroom, the closet, the dresser, chair, and any other items that are
for their individual use. If they are to have a roommate, introduce
them, tell them something about each other to make them feel at
ease. Any special safety features should be pointed out to them. As
soon as possible, take them for a tour of the nursing home. Introduce
them to all the personnel they meet. This new patient should become
especially familiar with all the auxillary services that are available
and the people in charge of them.

The first few days of a patient's stay in a nursing home are
critical. They will set the pattern for the entire stay. Care should be
taken not to overwhelm patients. If they are tired, let them rest, but
look in on them frequently. Too many details will overwhelm and
confuse elderly patients, especially if they are feeble. Concentrate on
the simple and essential matters first. Be sure to demonstrate on how
to summon the nurse if they need one. Check with patients on how
they want their personal belongings placed. Discuss with the patients and dietary director preferences and special needs. It will
mean much to patients if they are asked for their preferences.

Check to see whether patients are depressed. See that they do not
become emotionally upset. Do they know the rules of the nursing
home? Show them that administrators and the staff are their friends,
and that they are there to help them to be happy in their new home.

Summary of what Needs to Be Done for a New Patient

1. Make the patient comfortable in the room.
2. Check medications and put them in a box in the medicine
   cabinet.
3. Check the doctor's orders and transfer sheet.
4. Take all vital signs including weight, if possible.
5. Make out chart and other relative remarks.
6. Call doctor's office to notify him of patient's arrival. Check when
   he will come, and report this to the patient.

7. Check medication with the doctor if signed orders are not available.
8. Check treatments and special orders.
9. Check for medical history and diagnosis.
10. Make physical examination.
11. Prepare nameplates for identification.
12. Mark clothing, make list, and list valuables.
13. Notify dietary director, activities director, all special staff, and the laundry.
14. Make medication cards.

EVALUATION OF PATIENT'S NEEDS

It must be clearly understood that the evaluation of a patient who has just come into a nursing home is one of observation and careful examination by staff members in order to serve this patient in every way possible. The staff members do not take the physician's place but have the responsibility to treat the patient every day. Evaluation for treatment of the *whole person* is their aim.

Mental Evaluation

Evaluate the whole person:
1. Mental illness with organic symptoms.
2. Somatic illness as a mental disturbance.
3. Action of drugs on the patient.
4. Is the patient senile?
5. Does he talk coherently in answer to your questions?
6. Is he depressed because of his new surroundings?
7. Does he seem to be normal in his reactions?
8. Did he come from a normal home life?
9. Look into his background for answers to his feelings on coming to the nursing home.
10. Others, such as memory, reasoning, and emotions.

Physical Evaluation

1. Look at the patient's skin.
2. Is he tired? Does he tire easily?
3. Are there organic problems?
4. What is the diagnosis?

5. Look at the eyes. Can he see? Does he need glasses? If yes, how badly does he need them? Can he see without glasses; to what extent?
6. Is he in pain? Where does it hurt?
7. Check the pulse rate, temperature, respiration, and blood pressure.
8. How much exercise has been done in the past?
9. What is the customary diet? Quantity of food?
10. Are there any allergies to foods, clothing, soap, or other elements?
11. How are his teeth? Does he wear dentures? What about dental hygiene?

Social Needs

1. Is the patient accustomed to being with people? Does he come from a large family? Does the family live close by? Is the wife or the husband nearby? Who is the closest relative?
2. Who is responsible for finances?
3. Who is responsible for his entrance to the nursing home?
4. Does the patient sing or want to participate in social activities? Does he like to talk and participate or just watch? Has the director of activities talked to the patient? Can you help the director plan activities that this particular patient desires?
5. Does he like to read? Does the nursing home have a library where he can get books?
6. Will he be taken out of the home for visits?
7. What is he physically capable of doing?

Recreational Needs

An effective recreational director can assist in making the nursing home a place to live — not just a place to die. The ability to motivate, to be involved and enjoy life while recuperating, is equally important as a good nursing service. Little benefit is derived in rehabilitating a patient who sits with an idle mind, not enjoying life, not having much to look forward to except mere existence. A patient with proper motivation and a strong desire to live will respond more readily to medical treatment. The person who leads this program should be friendly, compassionate for the elderly, and sincere and should have a desire to make life more pleasant for the patients. To achieve these goals, the recreational director must be able to communicate with the patients.

1. Ascertain their likes and dislikes — what they enjoy doing.
2. Can and do they like to work with their hands? If they do, that opens the areas of arts, crafts, and painting.
3. Are they religious persons? If they are, then you have a need for church services and for participation with religious leaders in various activities.
4. If they read, then you should have a library and reading services with group discussions based upon the books read.
5. For those who are more physically capable, there are various games whereby the patients are with a group participating in physical activities.

The number of activities in a nursing home is only limited by the ability of its recreational director. Anything that the patients have an interest in becomes a part of the overall recreational program of a nursing home.

Family Relationships

The happiness of a patient, in many cases, depends on the attitude of the family and their relations to the patient. The administrator, upon first meeting the family, sets the pattern for the proper relationship between the patient, the family, and the nursing home. Thus, the first meeting must emphasize that this is the patient's home. If the family and patient sense this feeling, they immediately are on the administrator's side in helping the patient become a happier and better adjusted person in the new setting. The director of nursing must emphasize to the family that he is working with them and the patient's physician in trying to improve the patient medically.

The aides, who actually do the work with the patient, must be willing to discuss with the family the patient's likes and dislikes in the way he is treated. Where and how aides hang patients' clothes may be very important to patients. The tone of voice plays an important role in patients' attitudes. They respond very quickly, both pro and con, to the pitch of a staff worker's voice. Speak slowly, carefully, and distinctly.

Patients want to make friends because they are lonely in this new home. All of the staff personnel, in dealing with the family, have the responsibility of explaining the routine and activities that patients have available to them.

Many families have a guilt complex upon putting their loved ones into a nursing home. Thus, they are looking for some attitudes or activities to which they can object. Be sure to mention to the family that the dietary director not only looks at the chart for dietary instructions from the physician but also goes to the patient's room to discuss with the patient and family the needs for special foods and diets. The patient must be made a part of the society at the home as soon as possible to eliminate complaints from the family.

After the primary needs are met, the aged handicapped patient has other needs on which adjustment is based. Emotional security, relationships with other patients, and the sense of personal growth and worth are some of the extras that the patient seeks. These are essential for good mental hygiene, which is dependent on a satisfactory self-image, recreation, and good interpersonal relations. These elements are of basic importance for maintaining health and physical function and affect the quality of the patient's life and its duration.

These needs are related to the success of the purely medical aspect of rehabilitation. They affect motiviaton during the therapy, as well as the retention of gains once therapy is complete. Unless the physician is aware and concerns himself with the patient's adaptation to life, the physical gains that are made are apt to be relatively useless in the long run. Although a person in later life has acquired a disability, this does not, except in limited cases, deprive him of his human needs and satisfactions. Of course, his tempo and his goals are different from what they were at an earlier age. The medical profession does not yield to the temptation to assume that these needs and satisfactions can be ignored. If they are ignored, the possibility is greatly increased that the patient will deteriorate into a state of declining physical and mental health.

Each patient's needs and characteristics must be considered to determine his adjustment to life in a nursing home. These include such factors as personality and attitudes, his family structure and relationships, his housing and his economic background. Every person/patient has a different equation, which is made up of these elements in combination with his health and physical condition. He must be treated as a whole if his adjustment and health are not to suffer. The medical profession has come to realize that to confine its skills to the treatment of physical ills without a deep regard for the patient as a person with needs in many other areas is incomplete and unsatisfactory. Physicians have always been aware of the personalities of their patients, as well as their social and economic background, but have not brought this into true perspective with patients' needs. It is indeed true that the same physicians, although aware of the other factors, have totally ignored them because they were not medical problems per se.

Medical education is changing this concept, and nowhere is it more needed than in the treatment of the aged, disabled, chronically ill patient. The United States Health Survey estimated in July, 1967, that there were 756,239 people in 19,141 nursing homes. In 1977, it was estimated that there were 22 million people over the age of sixty-five and 1.2 million in nursing homes.

For those patients who must live in a nursing home, restorative services for physical and mental health must be available, or secondary complications will arise, which could make the person deteriorate into one that is sick and ready to die. The interdependence between a patient's physical needs and his attitudes and his emotions are important to the restoration of the person. In addition, one must keep in mind that a person's environment is closely related to the status of mind, body, and emotions.

COMMON SERVICES

Some thought must be given to rooms or areas that are used by all the patients at one time or another. If the facility is called a nursing home, these areas must make the resident/patient feel he is part of a communal society. Each area should have its own personality. Most important is privacy in the individual's rooms, and the communal rooms or areas should allow the resident/patient to share ideas and experiences with others. Living together, especially with strangers, requires adjustment and understanding. The common services and areas must be planned and coordinated to contribute towards this end. The needs of the individuals to be served must always be the factor determining the extent to which communal areas are planned. Some homes try to include facilities and plans to take care of the infirm and those that are ambulatory. It is axiomatic that the individual should give as well as receive.

If there is group communication, this will give the individual incentive to become part of a living community, as opposed to the deterioration to which continued privacy may lead. Architects may make their plans from books. In most cases, they are young and must be told the wants and needs of a nursing home. There must be an emphasis in common rooms on making them small and intimate, thus conveying privacy among activity. The proper arrangements of furniture, lights, and colors must give the feeling of warmth and togetherness. Safety features should be part of these areas. The living areas where most activities are carried out should have a lounge somewhere in the central part of the building to make it easily accessible to all residents/patients. There should be one or two smaller living communal areas close to the sleeping areas, making it convenient to go from one's room to this communal area. The main lounge can be used by larger groups for recreational purposes, such as films, plays, and parties. The smaller areas can be used by individuals and their visitors as well as small groups to share things together such as cards, chess, or just talk.

One other area that is used more than just any other space in a nursing home is the dining area. The decor of this room can make dining a pleasure and lead to good participation by all. It is desirable to have a screened area so that if there are patients who are embarrassed by how they eat, they can have some measure of privacy. The tables and chairs must be arranged so that people in wheelchairs and crutch walkers can pass between them. Furthermore, the tables should be made high enough to get wheelchairs under them. Visitors of patients/residents who wish to eat with the residents must be accommodated.

Some thought must be given to religious services for residents. If space is available, then a special area can be set aside for this; if not, then the main lounge or recreational room or dining area can be used for this purpose.

A nursing home must be flexible; the staff must keep in mind that continual changes must be made. Thus, as the types of patients/residents change, a nursing home must adapt or lose their patients. All of the preceding factors in planning and carrying out the function of a nursing home affect the physical and mental health of the patients. Success depends on the ability of a nursing home to adjust to the changes and to keep the patients happy.

THE NURSE AND NURSING SERVICE

The nurse who works with the elderly in a nursing home is someone special. One definition of nurse, found in the *Oxford Dictionary,* states the following: *"Nurse."* One who fosters, tends, cherishs, promotes the growth, and development or healing of a person."

This is the ideal of the geriatric nurse who performs nursing services for the care of the elderly. Nursing encompasses direct bodily care, the re-establishment of impaired mental or physical functions, and the maintenance or development of the patient's social ties with his family and friends. For most elderly patients with long-term disorders, the nursing home is home, and nursing the principal therapy. The increase in chronically sick people and expansion of medicine and its specialties have resulted in a decreased number of nurses available for general duty. This has caused a new class of people in the field of nursing care.

Responsibility for carrying out the orders of the physician has shifted from the registered nurse to the licensed vocational or practical nurse and to the aides. This has resulted in a breakdown in standards of nursing service. Patient care has suffered because less qualified people are carrying on the nursing service. One solution that has been initiated is to appoint a person to take care of the routine business and physical arrangements of nursing service and allow nurses to become teachers. They can teach lesser trained people and thus provide better patient care to elderly patients. One of the most important aspects of nursing care that the head nurse or director of nursing must assume as a governing principle will be to encourage the elderly patient to feel that he is a separate and distinct person — that he has a sense of control over his destiny, his right to be a member of the rehabilitation team with a voice to vote and even the power to say no. Nursing must foster, not stifle, individuals.

Most elderly patients respond to kindness, patience, understanding, and sensitivity. Understanding of their disability and their individuality is what they appreciate in those who work with them. It does not matter whether the staff members are registered nurses, licensed practical or vocational nurses, nurses' aides, or others from the rehabilitation team; they want your understanding. The attitude of the director of nursing, who is also usually the head of the rehabilitation team and the key person, is important to a successful team effort. If nurses deal with patients as people rather than a diagnosis, these feelings will filter down to the staff and other professionals. If the head nurse or director of nursing encourages the staff to get to know the patients, their likes and dislikes, their present and past physical and emotional conditions, their family background, the type of work they did, the way they happened to come to the nursing home, their expectations for improving their condition, and the means by which they plan to achieve some success in activities of daily living, the chances of the teams achieving their goals is greatly enhanced, and the result is better understanding between the patient and the staff.

It must be noted that in many nursing homes the head nurse or director of nursing may have one or two other registered nurses but no experts in the field of rehabilitation, no psychologist, no social worker, no physical therapist. The problem with this situation is that there are many patients to look after, and the director of nursing may have many nurses' aides and assistants who have had no formal training. As a result, the director must become a teacher and by instructions encourage the staff to work closely with each patient. The director must encourage these assistants to help the patients to achieve their goals. He must see that each patient has realistic goals in their physical, recreational, social, and mental areas. If the physician and the director of nursing give realistic goals, encouragement, individualized consideration, and genuine attention to each patient, not only may their attitudes lead patients to try and try again, but they will become behavioral models to auxiliary personnel who are as eager to see patients improve as the physician and the director of nursing. The head nurse and the physician must conduct in-service training programs for their staff. Reaching their goals can be very satisfying to both the patient and the staff. The basic attitudes of nursing to remember are: respect for the person and unconditional acceptance and stimulation of the patients' capacities to discover a way to live more fully.

The physician depends on nurses and staff to alert him to his patients' condition. Some danger signals that must be reported immediately are the following:

1. Acute pain in the eye. This could indicate glaucoma.
2. Sudden loss of vision. This could mean a detached retina.
3. Sudden loss of hearing. This could be caused by a vascular accident.
4. Infection. This is shown by a low grade of fever.
5. Upset stomach and indigestion.
6. Sudden blood loss.
7. Heartburn that persists for some time.
8. Marked changes in bladder and bowel movements.

The nuring service in a skilled nursing home should and must be under the direct control of a registered nurse with special training or interest in rehabilitation. Nursing services should be available on a twenty-four-hour basis. Medicare spells out in more detail their duties and responsibilities. Furthermore, if registered nurses are not on hand for direct supervision of patients on the basis, then it is their responsibility to see that a licensed practical or vocational nurse can perform those duties for them.

The latest trend in the area of nursing service is the development of a class of personnel called nurses' aides. These personnel have no training except their willingness to work for a wage. If the nursing home is willing to pay good or above average wages, they will get better quality personnel. By the same token, poor wages mean less qualified people, and the patient is the one to suffer. The nurses' aides render the most direct personal service to the patient — the key area for teaching and in-service training. The ability of the director of nursing to prove that he is capable of inspiring these individuals to give the best care possible is of utmost importance.

PSYCHOSOCIAL ASPECTS OF REHABILITATION

Health Manpower

The health delivery system is classified as an industry and, as such, is the third largest in the national economy and is growing rapidly. A listing of health occupations by primary title adds up to

121 types; by secondary titles, the total is 246. Given this data, it is no surprise that territorial rights and struggles for status, licensure, accreditation, and certification assume so much importance in the health care field. In the field of rehabilitation, the following classifications of allied health personnel are listed:

Physical therapists
Occupational therapists
Speech therapists
Hearing therapists
Prosthetic technicians
Social workers

Health Services Personnel

One result of the knowledge explosion has been a corresponding increase in classifying health personnel by the specialized knowledge and skills important to health care activities. Most are classed under the heading *allied health professions* largely because this term is used in federal documents. Are they professionals?

One definition of a profession that is most apt is the one that Supreme Court Justice Brandeis gave: "A profession is an occupation for which preliminary training is intellectual in character involving knowledge and learning as distinguished from mere skill, which is pursued largely for others and not merely for one's self." One can add that the professional spirit of service requires a willingness to sacrifice time.

In 1962, the Eastman Kodak Company's advertisement in a leading professional magazine was addressed to the concept of professionalism. It contains the essence of the goals of a professional person, and the means to achieve them.

1. Professionalism and chance have little in common.
2. Professionalism is experience, the total of it. Like a bank account, it grows upon deposits, year upon year deposits with all the sacrifices of investment of self.
3. Professionalism is competence to perform regardless of convenience, fatigue, or luck.
4. For the true professional, the better he becomes, the higher the standard.
5. Each patient depends upon medical professionalism, skill long

practiced, experience long ready, and standards long honored.

The personnel of the nursing home consist of the registered nurses, the licensed vocational and practical nurses, the nursing aides, the dietary help, the maintenance help, and all the professional specialists. All these people influence the elderly patient of the nursing home. We will discuss the various specialists in the field, we will study the patients' problems, their emotional and physical problems, their reactions to their handicap and the ways to motivate them to try to achieve their goals. It is time we took into consideration the interactions between the patients, the medical personnel, the nursing staff and all the other people who actually have contacts with the patients. All of the specialists in the field deal with their areas for a short period of time each day. The physician makes his visit, the nurse gives the patient his medications and does the dressing, but that leaves most of the care for the day to the supportive personnel who work the eight-hour shifts. There is a great need for all the specialists to gain the wholehearted support, understanding, and cooperation of the supportive personnel. There must be a method made to communicate with this group. Professionals must try to understand and study them for rehabilitation to succeed. Without their help, very little success can be achieved by the specialist and the patient.

In general, we study patients' physical disabilities, their particular needs, the degree of their handicap, their personalities, their psychosocial situation, and their places in the nursing home. We recognize that many times a physical disability has been aggravated by their psychological problems. The treatment plan made by the rehabilitative team must gather data concerning the nature and the degree of the handicap along with the nature of its psychological stress on the patient. The patient's degree of adjustment is a key factor in the program to be made.

We can all understand that nearly all patients experience a degree of shock and disbelief at the onset of a serious illness and usually show signs of withdrawal, grief, anxiety, or anger as they become aware of its severity and perhaps realize the long time it will take to recover, if at all.

A team is a group of people who are working together to help a patient become rehabilitated. If all of these members do their jobs and if they work together, they are successful in their goals for a particular patient. All members of the staff are specialists. They are experts in nursing, physical therapy, occupational therapy, social service, speech and hearing therapy, dietary services, recreation, psychological services, and practicing medicine. The physician in a long-term patient care makes the initial diagnosis and evaluation. Then, if he is a good leader, he turns the whole rehabilitation over to these experts. He acts as a liaison, or leader or captain, who plays a part only when needed. He deals with medical problems. This leader must delegate much of his authority of treatment decisions to the staff, relying upon the skills of the members of the team to determine goals and therapeutic tactics. At all times the team that many patients require a relationship with a person who will be with them many hours a day actively working with them in their efforts to get well. Each patient will pick a different member of the team to share their lives, so to speak, during their period of rehabilitation or convalescence. If the team develops a true spirit of cooperation, it is reflected in their work. Patients who are keenly sensitive to the people who work with them realize that they have a group of friends who are experts all working with them. One big problem in team efforts occurs when the majority of people work together but one or two members pull in another direction. If this happens, the physician must step in and make a decision either to get the team together or to break up the team and have the staff members who have the most realistic goals work with the patient in question.

People who are willing to listen can learn to know their handicapped elderly patients/residents because usually these people are starved for conversation. Patients enjoy talking to someone who will listen. Some patients may have a short attention span, or they may have some difficulty with speech, but the person working with them has numerous opportunities to talk to them, e.g. when bathing them, helping them get dressed, or assisting them in eating. Too often we speak of lack of communication between staff and member of the rehabilitation team, but more often there is a lack of communication with the patient. It is up to the specialist to start the communication chain from the patient to the highest level of administration.

Another area that needs staff's attention is understanding that most people do not like to change. Patients have established a routine with which they are happy. The aged patient with handicaps has especially developed a set pattern, a routine. Each day the habits of yesterday become more fixed. Those who work with these patients must recognize that it takes time to get the aged patient to change. Think of how much of a shock it must be for elderly patients to leave their homes and families and come to a nursing home. They suddenly are with strangers. In many cases, they have no privacy; someone else shares a room with them. All of their prized possessions are left behind. They are bewildered and lost, and now people want to change their daily routines. One of the things the staff can do to lessen the shock is by allowing patients to have some of their things from home with them.

An example of leaving some routine intact could be the patient's habit of brushing his teeth or cleaning his dentures at a certain time, the place he stores his dentures at night. Why change these habits when it does not interfere with his disability but it does help him emotionally? If patients have been lying in bed most of the day at home and now the staff is trying to get them ambulatory, they need encouragement to get up. They must have a reason, such as, "You will feel better sitting up to eat." Staff members may want them to visit another patient whom they know or to go to an activity that they say they enjoy. Patients who learn to do things for themselves are happiest. Therefore, staff members encourage their patients to learn to do all everyday living activities.

If there is good communication from patient to nurse or nurses' aide, to the therapists of the rehabilitation team, to the physician, then to the family, everyone knows the patient's capabilities, achievements, and goals.

It is essential to remember that in taking care of elderly patients the purpose is to help restore them to the fullest possible degree of mental, physical, and emotional health. Achieving these objectives may take more time and patience and may be interrupted for various reasons, but it can be reached.

HEALTH OF PERSONNEL

The health of the people who work in nursing homes is important. Most homes have a full-time maintenance department whose primary job is to see that the equipment used in the nursing home is in good repair. They also do a certain amount of preventive maintenance and general work to keep everything functioning. Yet, who looks after the health of the people who work in the nursing home? From the administrator to the lowest paid employee, it is the individual's responsibility to take care of his own health. Health is fundamental to good work — good health is reflected in good work, and poor health in poor work. The health of employees is directly related to their proficiency, dependability, quality of work, attitude, safety, and relationships with fellow workers. Health problems of employees comprise the entire list of human needs; thus, the administrator must be constantly alert to review the employees' records for evidence of any medical problem. A periodic health examination should be required.

It is the administration's responsibility to protect the health of the employees by instituting high safety standards. According to federal law under the Occupational Safety and Health Act, the administrator must see that work policies require the safest working conditions: proper heat and ventilation, safety equipment, good lighting, rest breaks, time for lunch, Health protection requires a review of the work program, job requirements, working conditions, safety, and infection control. There must be a program of education in health and hygiene, provision for first-aid and emergency medical attention, and a policy of sick leave and sick pay. Health services include employer's liability insurance, medical and health insurance, periodic health checkups, dental and optical services, guidance and counseling, and family services such as maternity leave for the working mother.

The issue of drugs and their ready availability to nursing home employees has made this a major health hazard.

The administrator today cannot take the health of his employees lightly, it is very important in the success or failure of his nursing home. Its importance cannot be overemphasized.

The personnel of a nursing home should be adquate to carry out the aims and objectives of the nursing home and its patients. The following staff members absolutely needed:

1. A physician who is knowledgeable, up-to-date, and interested in geriatrics.
2. A director of nursing who is rehabilitation minded or trained.

3. An administrator who is trained and wants only the best for his patients.
4. A director of recreation and activities.

Other staff members to add, if this is possible, are the following:

1. A physical therapist
2. An occupational therapist
3. A dietitian
4. A social worker, on call
5. A speech therapist, on call
6. A psychologist, on call

The preceding staff must consider the following factors in the determination of the degree of supervision that their patients need:

1. Mental evaluation of patients: The degree of confusion, memory impairment, disorientation.
2. Degree of mobility: The ability of patients to ambulate and aids the need.
3. The amount of self-care: The ability to dress, to feed self, use of toilet, and all the activities of daily living.

It is an accepted fact that one of the biggest problems that confronts the administration of a nursing home is getting and keeping a good staff. The recuitment, selection, and placement of the staff is a very important function. It is one of the administrator's prime functions. If he gets a good staff, then the success of his administration is assured. Locating properly qualified personnel is a hard and, at times, a very discouraging process. The interviews with prospective employees requires tact and skill. The purpose of the following pages is to give some suggestions on practices that are necessary after the staff has been hired, namely, on-the-job training, in-service training, and other facets of employee relationships.

In the typical nursing home setting the team is very small. They are composed of the physician, who may come once a week, or twice a month, once a month, or when called; the director of nursing, who sees the patients, as they enter the home; the charge nurse; the dietitian; the licensed vocational or practical nurse; and the aides. In some cases, there is a specialist, i.e. physical therapist, either on the staff or as a consultant, a recreational therapist, or activities director. A speech therapist and a psychologist might also be used as consultants. In some cases if it is impossible to get a physical therapist, an occupational therapist will be consulted. However, the members of the team with the most influence with the patients are the aides. They work with the patients twenty-four hours a day and, thus, are the people who influence the lives of the patients more than any other members of the rehabilitation team. Unfortunately, in many cases they are the least trained in rehabilitation, and the least paid. They are often unhappy because they are not listened to and not appreciated by the professionals; they cannot make a decision concerning their patients without getting prior approval from someone with more authority. Only when members of the rehabilitation team work together and respect each other can they make a success of the objectives.

It has been the author's experience that if the leader of the rehabilitation team takes the proper approach to the staff team, they will give him their wholehearted support. Furthermore, this group is starved for further learning. They will benefit from in-service training and on-the-job training.

THE PATIENT AND THE PERSONNEL

The patients as a group in a nursing home situation are unique. Unfortunately, the staff seldom listen to them. For some reason beyond reason, too many of the staff, whether they are professionals or paraprofessionals in the medical field, do not like the patients to tell them anything. It might be a reflection of a sense of inadequacy at the inability to cure these handicapped individuals and to cope with their anger toward these failures. Yet, patient groups can provide a significant benefit to each member of the team by supporting each member's attempt at rehabilitation. Patients are interested in their program and should be listened to for suggested changes that might give some better chances for success. Such patient-staff groups demand an exceptional mutual confidence and communication, and it may well be the approach for the future. By meeting frequently with the patients as groups, the staff has an opportunity to take the therapeutic advantage of the group process. Rather than talking about the terrible food or about each other, the patient groups can assume a certain amount of responsibility in many functions of the treatment plan.

In most cases this is so unusual and contrary to the traditional concept of the patient as a passive recipient of medical attention that personnel and programmers are very slow to take advantage of the patient group process by becoming a part of it.

The Joint Commission on Accreditation of Nursing Care Facilities and Residential Care Facilities points out the following:

> There shall be evidence in writing of acceptable administrative policies, practices, and procedures. There shall be prepared administrative manuals explaining patient/resident care policies and procedures in regard to admissions, discharges, refunds, and other pertinent information relating to the total operation of the facility. Responsible persons shall be informed periodically regarding the condition of the patient/resident and notified in the event of an emergency change in the patient/resident status. There should be two (2) or more licensed doctors of medicine who shall agree in writing to advise on medical-administrative problems, review the institution's program of patient care, provide for utilization review, and handle emergencies if the individual's personal physician is unavailable.

WRITTEN POLICIES AND PROCEDURES

Nursing homes today provide a wide variety of specialized services and activities in addition to many of the basic services. As nursing home institutions become more complex, as they offer a greater variety of services, more decisions must be made by more people. The further down in the organizational structure the decision is made, the more guides that are needed to help them make an appropriate decision. Established policies and procedures in written form provide these needed guides. Thus, the purpose of established policies and procedures, in written form, is to provide guidelines to assist nursing homes to establish their policies and procedures.

All organizations have policies and procedures. They are important for decision making and efficient management. Those who benefit from such written policies and procedures are the following:

1. The administration staff
2. The physician
3. The employees
4. The general public
5. The patients

The administrator has a means of control when there are stated policies in written form. It helps the morale of supervisors because they have something definite on which to base their decisions. Their authority is stated, and they know that their supervisors will uphold their decisions because it is based on written policy. Another advantage is that during the process of putting these policies and procedures into written form one may discover areas that no policy or procedure has ever been made. Thus, gaps are closed. One can also identify overlapping areas and duplications.

Nursing homes deal with insurance companies and city, county, state, and federal agencies. They all look at how the institution is run. They have certain requirements, and they want to see if the nursing home's standards match theirs.

For example, one of the conditions for participation in Medicare is, "The governing body is responsible for implementing and maintaining written policies and procedures that adequately support sound patient care." Thus, in order to qualify for payment, to obtain and retain a license, and to receive accreditation, written policies and procedures are a necessity.

Written policies and procedures can be used in —

1. employees' handbooks;
2. orientation;
3. in-service training;
4. public relations;
5. administrative handbook.

Following are some ideas for the contents of these different handbooks:

1. The employees' handbook would include personnel policies, work regulations, benefits, services to be performed.
2. The orientation handbook would contain material that will serve to inform all employees of the function and duties of their particular job or position.
3. The in-service handbook would give employees information concerning materials that will be used for continuing education on the job in order to improve their abilities.
4. The public relations handbook might include the policies and procedures for giving out information to special community organizations.

A pamphlet to get volunteers to help in the institution is another area of public relations. Pamphlets for physicians stating the nursing home's policies and standards will give them information concerning the institution that they did not know. The patient care program or rehabilitation program will be of special interest to physicians if they have need for such special services.

Development of Policies and Procedures

Policies are classified as (1) general administrative and (2) service or departmental

1. General Administrative Policies: These affect the majority of the operations of the institution. They include personnel and many other policies that cross departmental or service lines, such as admission policies.
2. Services or Departmental Policies.
   a. Apply to only service or department; an example would be the nurse's giving out medications.
   b. Patient care policies; these would range from medication, food service, physical therapy treatments, financial arrangements, for special services not provided by the nursing home, e.g. dental care.

Policy gives direction for action. Procedure gives step-by-step instructions in how the action is to be carried out. It is suggested that an advisory group to help in setting policies and procedures be composed of professional and administrative persons whose experience and training makes them competent to evaluate patient care and needs of the institution. Procedures are the "how" of operations. They should be determined by the people who are responsible for carrying them out. For example, nursing procedures should be determined by the director of nursing in conjunction with supervisors and other nursing personnel. Each department or service should work out its own procedure.

Suggested Procedure

The governing authority of an institution states a policy that patients in that institution will receive rehabilitation services of a certain quality and in the amounts consistent with the patient's needs.

The administrative staff consisting of the administrator, the director of nursing, and the physician plan the rehabilitation program. This is related to the physician's orders concerning patients' needs. This becomes the policy of the institution after the highest authority of the nursing home has approved it. Now procedures can be written implementing them. For example, nursing service policy states that medication is to be given at the hours specified by the physician. The procedure will then state exactly who in the nursing personnel is responsible.

CONTENTS OF POLICY AND PROCEDURE PAMPHLET.

1. History and background of the institution:
   People are interested in the background of places in which they work. Employees take pride in telling their friends about where they work. Suggested items that might be included are as follows:
   a. Date when the institution founded
   b. Who founded it
   c. The reason it was founded
   d. Other locations
   e. Bed capacity
   f. Type of institution
   g. Future plans for the institution
2. Goals of the institution:
   Goals should express the desired results toward which the institution is working. Goals may be expressed idealistically in terms of the results hoped for or they can be expressed realistically in terms of what accomplishments can actually be expected.

GOVERNMENT SUPPORT OF NURSING HOME-CARE

In the past seven years, Congress has recognized three kinds of nursing homes: (1) skilled nursing homes, (2) extended care facilities, and (3) intermediate care facilities.

Medicare currently pays for well over one-half of all nursing home services in the country. Improvements are being made in nursing home service, and quality varies in different homes. Governmental financing of nursing homes has focused special attention on deficiencies. Since the aged patient has no power to change conditions, it rests with the federal government to set standards for the inmates of the nursing homes.

In 1950, the Congress, by an amendment to the Social Security Act, authorized direct payments to providers for services in health care. In 1965, Congress created Medicare and called nursing homes certified to participate in Medicare *skilled nursing homes.* Today, Medicare payments for care in these skilled nursing homes amounts to almost half of all nursing home care in the country. Under Medicare, states are responsible for inspecting and certifying as skilled nursing homes institutions meeting state licensure standards and federal medical standards.

In 1965, Congress, under Medicare, recognized another nursing care facility called the *extended care facility.* Virtually all people sixty-five years of age and older are eligible to receive posthospital care. Nursing homes approved by Medicare are for the indigent over sixty-five years of age and in some cases for the medically indigent patient under welfare and Medicaid.

Total government spending for skilled nursing home care under Medicare is four times greater than for care in extended care facilities. Yet, extended care facilities under Medicare serve more patients per year at lower per capita cost. This represents a far more direct interest by the federal government in the extended care facilities.

The government under the Department of Health and Human Services has now set standards for national quality controls over nursing homes and extended care facilities. This attempt is prticularly important because the states have failed to provide adequate and uniform standards through their own licensure laws. The federal standards are designed not only to improve care but also to reorient it. In particular, they attempt to strengthen relations of nursing homes with hospitals and to emphasize rehabilitative services as opposed to custodial care.

There is no doubt that there is a need for improvements in most nursing homes today. There are many studies that indicate a high rate of serious diseases and disabilities in nursing homes due to the age of the patient/resident.

The first step toward improving the care of a patient in a nursing home would be to have the physician serve as the medical director for the nursing home. His duties should be specific and detailed about the care given by the staff of the nursing home. He can insure that the home maintains proper patient records, safety precautions, and overall services. Overall services should include nursing services, social services, nutritional services, psychological needs, and all phases of rehabilitation. He should periodically conduct in-service training programs and attend staff meetings. If there are nursing homes that cannot hire a physician, then the government, through the United States Public Health Service, should furnish a physician.

Another method for getting physicians for nursing homes would be to use medical school students, interns, and residents. Under the guidance of their teacher, they could treat patients in the hospital and upon discharge follow them into the nursing home to continue their treatment.

ORIENTATION

Orientation is an organized effort to acquaint the new employee with his job. Each person with whom the new worker is to have some association should be properly introduced. This is the first thing done by all supervising personnel in every department. This orientation will allow the new employee to learn the function and responsibilities of each area of a nursing home. For the orientation of a new employee who is to work in the dietary department, the supervisor of this department will carry out the same plan as the supervisor of nursing does with one of his new employees. Duties of the orientation supervisor might include the following:

1. Introduction and welcome by nursing home staff
2. Showing where personnel items are stored
3. Location of restrooms and employee lounge
4. Facilities for eating
5. Review of personnel policies
6. Use of the time clock
7. Introduction to their work group
8. Tour of the nursing home and their place to work
9. Safety rules in the use of special equipment
10. Safety rules in the handling of patients
11. Parking rules
12. Fire drill

13. Briefing concerning their department.

In discussing the work required, they will first receive on-the-job training, later they will participate in in-service training programs. If there is a regular plan outlined for this program, this material should be furnished at this orientation period. The new employees will be given a copy of the personnel policy booklet of the nursing home. This personnel policy should include the following items:

1. The person they talk to for information concerning their job
2. The nursing home's statement of objectives
3. Working hours, overtime pay
4. Holidays, rest periods, and time off
5. Benefits, insurance, hospitalization, pension plans, and others
6. Sick leave, leave of absence, extended leave
7. Vacation and requirements for eligibility
8. Safety rules
9. The pay period and pay day
10. Rules of conduct
11. Liability of the employees
12. Miscellaneous information

A job description must be given to the new employee with explanation of how this description was arrived at, i.e. supervisor, former employees, and administrator who all helped in formulating this job description. Included in this job description would be the following:

1. Explanation of the job — the various responsibilities and duties.
2. Duty schedule.
3. List of place or places the job is to be accomplished, such as source of supplies, the check in and the check out stations.
4. Skills and techniques needed to do the job. Discussion of the necessary tools and equipment needed for the job.
5. The need for this job.
6. Title of the job.
7. The scope of the job.
8. The normal position and place the work is to be done.
9. The ways the job relates to other members of the staff.

ON-THE-JOB TRAINING

The purpose of on-the-job training is nothing more than teaching employees to do their job better, because doing a better job means better service. Improved service means the patient benefits. It also means employees get more satisfaction out of doing their jobs.

In the old days, on-the-job training was called an apprenticeship. Apprentices received formal instruction, and they also actually did the work under the supervision of an experienced worker. The idea of apprenticeship is based upon the ability of the experienced worker to guide new employees in learning to perform their skills in a proper manner.

In some cases, formal training is also involved. A definite course of study in a classroom in the nursing home is given for one or more new employees from the same department. The length of time for on-the-job training varies with the personnel. The experienced worker and the ability of the new employee are the factors that determine the length of time required. A plan for on-the-job training should include the following:

1. Description of the training schedule
2. Reason for the training program
3. Objectives or purpose of the program
4. Outline of program
5. Any aids, books, and other material needed for training

Suggested Method

First, there should be formal instruction and demonstration. Then the trainee starts work on the job. A plan must be developed to teach each function of the job analysis, or description of the position. Therefore, each task must be broken down into its separate parts. Each task is then demonstrated by the experienced worker, and then the new employee or apprentice practices doing it. Sufficient time must be allowed for mastering each step before proceeding to the next. The demonstrator should progress from the simple tasks to the more difficult. The amount of detail needed to define a task is related to the type of task and the experience or lack of experience of the learner.

Naturally, the teacher will assume that the experienced employee already has working skills and needs merely a demonstration of methods used by the particular nursing home and an evaluation of his level of skill. The inexperienced employee will need a detailed explanation of each task and adequate practice. There are a number of basic functions performed in the nursing home that belong in a patient care manual which could serve as the basis for on-the-job training. Some tasks such as bed making, positioning, ambulation, medical asepsis, serving and feeding, personal care, skin care, admission and discharge, charting, vital signs, collecting specimens, etc. will be in the patient care manual.

There should be periodic checkups on the work done by new employees, perhaps at the end of the first week and then at least once a month. In cases where new employees are learning a new phase of their work, there should be a checkup at the end of each phase.

MOTIVATION

Motivation asks the question, Why do people act the way the do? It is important to motivate people because workers in a nursing home deal with people. To rehabilitate people, one must get them to want to do something. Also, the employees of a nursing home need to be motivated to to what they are hired to do. Psychologists point out that there are two basic needs that motivate people: (1) the need to belong and (2) the need for self-preservation.

Employees are motivated by the following:

1. The working conditions. They are people who have likes and dislikes, beliefs, goals, ideals, and needs. The place of employment and the conditions under which they work will encourage or discourage them. If the nursing home is clean, odorless, and sanitary, it will affect the employee's mental attitude, and they will respond more willingly to work.
2. Having a lounge.
3. Having a scheduled break.
4. Privileges relating to personal problems.
5. Work security. This is very important to employees. They want steady employment with an opportunity for promotions. They prefer a regular vacation and are concerned with sick leave and

fringe benefits. If the employees are satisfied that they have a good job, they will have a greater incentive to develop reliable work habits.

Workers like to take pride in their work and will respond when good quality work is expected of them. Employees that are free to excel and improve will find motivation to work.

In a nursing home where new ideas are respected and used, the employees usually come to work more eagerly. Employees do best at things they like to do. If they care, they are proud of their work.

It can be said that to get good motivation, workers must have —

1. a good working environment;
2. good supervision;
3. respect of fellow workers;
4. a job they like;
5. a job that promises security;
6. a challenging assignment.

Further thoughts on motivation bring up the all-important factor of recognition, which is one of the key factors. Workers also appreciate consideration. If employees make a mistake, they should be informed in such a manner that it does not turn them away from the administrator. The administrator must be considerate of their feelings and make them want to improve in order to get approval. In the area of consideration and recognition should be included giving people credit for the good things they are doing. Recognize the good as well as the bad and give due recognition to both. Remember, workers want the approval of their boss, whether it is the supervisor or the administrator. They want to be friendly with their supervisor and yet they want to respect him. Remember that recognition in the form of increased pay is a sure way of proving the sincerity of praise.

IN—SERVICE TRAINING

To have a successful nursing home it is important to have a required training program. There are always new methods, techniques, and equipment coming out that will help workers to do their jobs easier and better. The program must be well planned to be effective. It should be for all employees.

Goals

The administrator must make a survey of the nursing home's training needs. Is the performance good? Is the home full of patients? Are there any supervisory problems? Others? Factors that need to be considered are the following:

1. Problems
2. Performance
3. Communications
4. Equipment utilization
5. Skills
6. Supervision
7. Personnel and its organization
8. Operation
9. Procedure
10. Attitudes
11. Others

Overcoming identified needs becomes the goal of a training plan. Goals must be specific. They must be written and then broken down from goals into specific objectives. Once goals and objectives are set, the next step is choosing the supervisor and the location for this training to take place.

Supervisor and Place of Training

The success of a training program depends upon the supervisor. This person must be knowledgeable, enthusiastic, well liked, respected, and dynamic. He must have some training in teaching and its techniques and, above all, must have the backing of the administration.

The administration members must work very closely with the supervisor in making their plans for the training. At this time, an important question comes up: Where should this training take place? So often good plans are laid, but the setting and environment is not conducive to learning. Too often, it will be held in a vacant patient room, where there are limited space and limited facilities. What is needed is a training room on the premises of the nursing home, which is equipped with facilities and equipment that the workers use in their everyday duties. This room may have mutiple uses such as the day room or a classroom. A certain section could be set aside for training and equipment could be kept there. Cabinets for storage, a blackboard, and other aids that are needed could be kept here. Another advantage to having a designated place for training is that the employees realize the importance of training to the administration — they are willing to give up this space for it. Furthermore, this room is available for the use of employees who wish to better themselves by going there during their time off, or leisure period, to seek any special knowledge that will help them do a better job.

Methods of Training

There are various methods that can be used in the training program. One method is personal instruction and training classes. These should be supported and enriched by seminars, guest speakers, demonstrations, and discussion periods.

To evaluate the success of training programs, the trainer must give oral, written, and demonstrative tests. Learning takes place if the following elements are present: the learner is interested in the learning situation, the learner is exposed to knowledge, the learner has the right attitude, the learner gains understanding, and the learner can apply his new knowledge.

If teachers can include the following elements in their techniques, they will get the results desired, namely, a better equipped and knowlegeable worker who will make the nursing home outstanding:

1. Lecture
2. Discussion
3. Demonstration
4. Panel of experts
5. Tests
6. Workshops with small discussion groups
7. Seminars; directed study by small groups
8. Personal study and research assignments
9. Field trips to other nursing homes or hospitals
10. Visual aids
11. Audio aids

12. Forums; a speech, then a discussion

Training Aids

Four types of training aids are (1) films, (2) filmstrips, (3) slides, and (4) transparencies. It is important that if these aids are used the leader review them thoroughly because not all of the material can be used for every learning situation, nor will it always further the trainer's goal. A film can have its learning value increased by a proper introduction, noting certain points for the class to watch and discussing them at the end of the film.

Slides are becoming very popular because anyone with a good camera can take one. Especially effective is using a student or a patient for the slide. This makes for better attention to the slide, and it becomes a learning situation; they can see themselves actually doing the work.

Problems With Training Programs

When the administrator, the supervisor, the location, and the equipment are ready, the problem becomes when to program training. How can training be fit in a busy seven-day week and twenty-four-hour-a-day duty? Unless the administrator makes a definite schedule and follows it, success for training is quite limited. How can training be scheduled to use the largest percent of staff available? It is obvious that one cannot get 100 percent of the staff at one time for training. Therefore, it comes down to priorities, that is, scheduling and getting supervisors to cooperate. The administrator and the supervisor of training must set up a pro rata schedule for each section and see that the remaining workers take care of the patients while the others get their training.

The administrator is the key to the success or failure of the training program by motivating employees by showing them that this has top priority. Education is hard to sell, since it requires work above and beyond the duties listed. Too many employees feel that they know enough or that they are too old to learn or that they do not have the time.

Evaluation of the Program

One way to judge the success of the training program is by tests.

There are various types of testing available:

1. True and false statements or questions
2. Completion questions
3. Multiple choice questions
4. Essays
5. Oral testing
6. Observation of techniques
7. Interviews

Starting the Program

The administrator can make an announcement concerning the program either at a staff meeting or by posting a notice on the bulletin board where announcements are made to the staff. He will have to set up in written form his policies concerning the training program, definite assignments of time, place, and personnel in charge of the program. In many cases, the supervisors have been working on the details of the program, and in small nursing homes everyone knows what is happening. Make a big event out of the first meeting with pictures and announcements and perhaps get a local expert who is recognized in the field to make the first lecture-discussion program. The administrator should plan to attend and support the program.

HUMAN RELATIONS

Service is the primary function of the nursing home. The employees of this home are parties to this function; therefore, there must be a close relationship between management of the nursing home and its employees if a nursing home is to carry out its primary function. Naturally, all nursing homes have problems. In many cases, the first to be involved can solve the problem — the employee who deals directly with patients. This person who is closest to the conflict is in a position either to solve a problem or to bring it to the attention of the person who can solve it. This leads to communications between workers, supervisors, and administrator.

The lack of communication is a direct cause of problems' becoming so big that they cannot be solved. The problem must be relayed to someone who can solve it. Communication affects the exchange of information. The worker who first noticed the problem conveys his knowledge to the person he thinks can solve the problem. If this person cannot, the worker then conveys the information to another who is in a position to solve the problem. One must remember to give all the facts and observations so that there is a clear understanding in order to arrive at the best solution. Also, there is a need to have free exchange of ideas to arrive at a solution.

Another factor that must be considered in human relations is an element that causes a great deal of problems, and that is the relationship between departments. For example, there is very little direct relationship between nursing service and the housekeeping department because these two departments have very little in common; yet, they are dependent on each other. If maintenance does not keep the patients' rooms clean and the bathrooms working, how can nursing service go about the activities of daily living? It behoves the directors and supervisors of both of these services to have free communication as part of commitment to solving problems.

There must be a definite chain of command implemented in the daily work orders that is clear and easy to understand. The administrator can improve the relationship between departments. One of the best methods is to unify the supervisory staff. This can be done by scheduling activities that will bring them together. Once they get together to talk, think, and plan, their cooperation is stimulated. Another method could be in the training program. When workers learn together, there is increased opportunity for harmony and understanding.

Employee Morale

The morale of the employees is a key factor in a successful nursing home. If the morale is low, then problems never seem to get solved. The administrator who is cognizant of his employees' morale and makes an effort to do something about it will have a successful operation.

Following are suggestions for improving morale:
1. There must be a feeling of togetherness. All realized that they are equal members of a team that is trying to win. All recognize each others parts and know that together they can have a suc-

cessful operation.

2. Try to eliminate the factors that defeat morale.
   a. There may be a need to replace a supervisor or a person in a department who is always griping about something.
   b. Some of the activities that a particular department has to carry on, which they feel others should do, can be studied and changed if necessary for improvement.
   c. Some rules of the personnel department may be causing unrest.
3. Plan activities to increase morale, such as recognition awards, social activities, programs that will stimulate and improve relationships between employee and administration.
4. Some factors hinder good morale:
   a. Lack of challenging work
   b. Poor attitudes of leaders
   c. Fear of reprisal for making suggestions
   d. Unfair labor practices
   e. Classification of employees
   f. Lack of security

Successful administrators must be constantly on their toes to have a good nursing home. One of the requirements of the administrator is to be creative and have a good imagination. Serving the infirm, the aged, and the handcapped is a gigantic job in proportion to the number of available employees. As the administrator improves the quality of service, he raises the standards and goals of his nursing home. As the employees find themselves proud of their achievements, they also find that they have improved their own working conditions.

Creativity and imagination are functions of the mind. Each person stores his experiences, thoughts, knowledge, and beliefs in his mind. These can come from many sources such as work habits, reading, training, school, friends, etc. The more experience an employee is exposed to in the nursing home, the greater he builds his resources. Assimilating new experiences brings new information, which in turn causes formulation of new values. Persons looking for the solution must be very persistent in their search for it. Something must stimulate and motivate them to persist, and this applies to all the employees of a nursing home.

ETHICS

Ethics can be defined as practices and working relationships that are concerned with right and wrong. It has its source in beliefs, morals, goals, and attitudes towards one's profession. Ethics is related to a philosophy of life, a term used to describe thoughts and conduct. It is also related to morals and spiritual conduct. Social concepts and culture may define ethics to some extent. In the end, however, what one believes is right and what one believes is wrong will determine one's ethics.

Ethics is related to goals. To be ethical, goals must include a set of values, which in turn must be consistent with what is right. If we elevate standards of achievement, we also elevate ethics. This combination of factors is then translated into ethical practice.

Ethics in nursing care is the sum of the moral principles and practices necessary for proper care of the sick. Ethics is also an integral part of everyone's daily life, continually requiring the individual to make judgments of right and wrong and finally to decide how to govern personal conduct in keeping with these judgments. One's concept of ethics depends a great deal on the beliefs one has about humanity. An accepted premise in medicine is that man has control over his behavior, and it is this premise upon which ethical systems have been developed.

Basic Principles of Medical Ethics

Medical ethics is based on a belief in the moral obligations of those who work within the sphere of medicine. Those working in the health care services are under obligation to do the following:

1. Constantly maintain full professional knowledge of skills.
2. Safeguard the patient against danger to life and health and avoid unnecessary and unreasonable expense.
3. Observe professional secrecy and honor confidences disclosed in the process of treating the patient.
4. Refrain from engaging in illegal or immoral practices.
5. Safeguard the public and the professions from those who are deficient in moral character and competence. Ignorance and negligence are seen whenever a professional does not maintain a

standard of learning that enables him to have at his command the knowledge and techniques that improve his contribution to health care.

The health professional will not take risks in which a favorable outcome is highly doubtful. This professional must also honor confidence; if not, it could lead to awkward predicaments. A common problem in ordinary practice occurs when an unauthorized person insists on obtaining information about a patient. This problem arises often when someone inquires over the telephone about personal or medical problems of a patient. If the person's identity and his need for this information cannot be verified, deny it. Sometimes through careless conversation confidential information is given out. Even among members of the profession one cannot be careless concerning confidential information.

It behoves the members of a profession to police their own ranks in order to safeguard the public from those who are incompetent or morally deficient. It is an obligation to protect not only the public but also one's profession by maintaining the proper standards of a profession. A profession must never be compromised by the actions of a few. This detracts from the whole membership's image and status. This is a difficult problem for one who knows that one of his colleagues is incompetent. Usually the temptation is not to expose the incompetent — deciding to do so can be agonizing and calls for uncommon fortitude. However, failure to uphold the law and ethical codes is no less corrupt than their violation. In our society, wrongdoing is protested, and in doing so the law is upheld without fear of involvement or reprisal.

Public Relations

The reputation of the nursing home is what one might call its public image. Not only must it be spotless, but it must seem so to the general public. There is a difference. A nursing home may in fact be immaculate and give excellent service; however, it may have a poor public image because of an unpleasant past experience.

People contribute to the reputation of a nursing home. Every person who is associated with the home has input. Certainly the relatives and the patients form opinions and find many opportunities to reveal these opinions to the general public. The employees are another vital link with the public. Daily they demonstrate the home's character and personality, and the home is judged accordingly. Their talk, their honesty, their attitudes, their own general appearances speak constantly for, or against, the nursing home. The professional people who work with the patients may show willingness or unwillingness to recommend it on the basis of performance and policy. The business people who deliver supplies are spokesmen for the nursing home's atmosphere. The visitors tell others about their impressions of the nursing home services. Finally, the inspectors and regulatory personnel know perfectly well what the nursing home's image and reputation deserve to be.

The appearance of a nursing home makes a large difference in developing its image. The first impression is usually a lasting impression. Some people also get what might be called an aesthetic impression, which may be one of surprise or pleasure (this would be a positive impression) or unsightliness, smelliness, and general unsanitary conditions (this would be a negative impression). The general condition of the facility at any time will be the basis for the visitor's opinion.

Another important factor in the image of the nursing home could be the appearance of the patients themselves, and their attitudes. It is up to the administration, who is essentially the administrator, to be cognizant of all these factors to see that the first impression is a favorable one.

The administrator, in the final analysis, is the key to the success or failure of a nursing home. He is the leader in promoting public relations. The personnel that he picks, the persons to whom he delegates authority, the work practices of his staff, and the care given to the patients are all under his control. Furthermore, the employee relations are noticed by the patients and the public. If they are good, no one will notice, but if there have been labor troubles, everyone in the community will know it. This will be reflected in the public's opinion. The administrator is also the business head of the nursing home. The way he deals with businesses, his fairness, his honesty, and his promptness in paying bills all influence public opinion.

It is essential that the administrator be very conscious of his appearance, his dealings with others, and the home's appearance. He should never miss an opportunity to promote good will. He should participate in community affairs, as well as the affairs at the nursing home. He should live in the community. He can plan a low-key publicity campaign to focus attention on the variety of services offered by his nursing home.

The employees must be considered as the front line of public relations, for they are salesmen to the public. They are in direct contact with patients, family, visitors, professionals, and sales people. In fact, anyone who enters the nursing home comes in contact with the employees. What these employees do and how they act give people their first impressions of the nursing home. The employees must realize that anything they do in their personal lives reflects upon the home because the community associates their names with where they work. Therefore, the administrator must work with his employees to make them realize that they have a dual responsibility when they work for a nursing home. First, they must do a good job in the home for the patients, and second, they must conduct themselves in such a way in their personal lives that it reflects only good for the home. It would help the home if in the in-service training program, a section or a time were included for all employees to study the area of public relations. This would help the employees to realize the importance of their actions both in the home and when they leave.

The patient is the key to the assets of a nursing home's reputation. Each patient reflects the quality of care, attitudes, and the feelings of the staff of a nursing home. Patients generally talk to anyone who will listen. They talk to visitors, to their relatives, and to others who come into the home. Sometimes patients do not have to speak because their appearance speaks for itself. Hygiene, clothing, room, meals, and attitude are all a reflection of the home. Therefore, a good administrator can learn a great deal from his patients if he is willing to talk to them and listen to them. The administrator must try to make friends with all of his patients, which may not always be possible. He should make the effort, however, if he is to know what is going on in his home.

LAW AND THE PROFESSIONAL

Laws are essential to the harmony of all social groups in order to protect society and to regulate those activities which impinge on the rights of individuals and have the potential for harm. Liberty is not license. The first law of conduct must be self-discipline if man is to live fully. The discipline of formal law controls society's behavior and ensures orderly process of daily living. Laws define the obligations and benefits of prescribed behavior and also the penalties for not conforming to it.

In our society, there are regulations that are not specifically prescribed and enforced, but by the use of sanctions the members of a unit are informed if they do not conform. Through mores and taboos and expectation and understanding of what is acceptable conduct, social units maintain disciplining. Sanctions applied to those who do not comply include the withholding of approval and, in some cases, ostracism.

In the health field, there are laws that prescribed the limits of practice. These laws are usually spelled out in each state licensure law of a profession. On the whole, the physician usually remains legally resonsible for those who serve under his supervision. Interpretation of the law and its enforcement are in the hands of the courts of each political unit. The jurisdiction of the courts is determined by geography and by the types of cases to be tried.

Classification of Laws

1. Civil — negligence, libel, slander, commercial disputes, personal injuries.
   a. Contracts — agreements between person and organizations.
   b. Common law — principles, equity, rules of action.
2. Criminal.
   a. Misdemeanors — traffic violations, assault and battery; minor offenses.
   b. Felony — robbery, murder, arson, rape; serious offenses.
3. Martial — civil laws in times of emergency.
4. Military — for those in the armed forces who violate a law.
5. Statutory — violation of some state law, licensure, taxation, voting.

In the nursing home, the governing body is the legal agent of the home. This may be a corporation, it may be a charitable organization, and in some cases, it may be the legal entity of a city, town, or state. Usually the governing body gets a document that clearly states the institution's purpose and authority to function, which says —

1. that there will be the proper use of funds;
2. that there will be reasonable care and skill applied in the operation of the institution;
3. that the governing body will protect and preserve the property of the institution;
4. that satisfactory care for patients will be provided;
5. that due care and diligence in supervising the activities of the institution's personnel will be applied;
6. that a competent staff will be maintained.

The governing body may delegate these duties in appropriate manner with the proper authority to carry out the assignments, but this body is ultimately responsible before the law for the actions of those delegated.

In the past, the doctrine of immunity for charitable institutions and governmental institutions due to negligence of the hospital or its employees was upheld, but his has been changed in the recent years. Briefly, there are two types of liability in cases of negligence:

1. Respondent superior (let the master respond). The institution is responsible for the negligent acts of its employees.
2. Corporate negligence. Corporate liability applies to negligence associated with defective equipment, incompetent personnel, and poor maintenance of the building and grounds.

All employees of an institution, particularly professional personnel, must use every reasonable care in carrying out their duties. What is reasonable care? This is determined according to the standards common in that community by the same type of professionals. This is one reason why every institution must have rules and regulations that all employees must follow diligently.

Patient Consent

If the physician prescribes rehabilitation services, the specialist should discuss this with the patients and get their consent for these treatments or procedures. In some cases, not getting patients' consent could be viewed in the eyes of the law as commiting battery. It is essential that the professional person employed by an institution work within the limits of his professional competence. When he is asked to do something that he knows, or suspects, is outside the limits of his competence, he should, in order to protect himself from culpability if legal action is subsequently taken, state that his competency does not extend to this particular procedure.

1. Was there a medical order?
2. Was it written or oral?
3. Exactly what was given in that order?
4. Was it medically sound, and were the instructions complete?
5. If not, was the error or omission such that a reasonably competent professional person could be expected to question the order before carrying it out?
6. If it was sound and complete, did the person involved carry it out in a reasonably competent manner?
7. Was the accident unpredictable and unavoidable?

In view of these questions, there are a number of precautions that may be taken by people who are to carry out the order so that they will have maximum protection against culpability.

1. If the physician gives the order in person staff should —
   a. repeat it back to him before acting on it;
   b. remind him to write it on the patient's order sheet;
   c. check the order sheet after the physician leaves; if he forgets, make a note of the verbal order on patient's chart.
2. When the order is relayed by a second person —
   a. if it seems right, the staff should carry it out, then make note in patient's chart;
   b. if the staff have any doubts, they should contact the physician to verify order;
   c. if in doubt or cannot reach physician, they should check with their superior;
   d. if they feel the prescription is not appropriate, they should check with physician before giving treatment.

LICENSURE

The purpose of licensing professional personnel are as follows:

1. To discourage the growth of groups that claim the right to practice but whose members have not had proper education or training

2. To prevent nonqualified persons from calling themselves professionals
3. To allow reciprocity with those states which already have licensure or registration, so that professionals may move and practice without loss of legal status
4. To prevent any state from becoming a dumping ground for persons who cannot meet the standards of states requiring licensure or registration

The benefits of licensure are the following:

1. To the public — assurance of receiving competent services
2. To the health profession — availability of quality service
3. To the patient — protection against misrepresentation by nonqualified persons.

PATIENTS' BILL OF RIGHTS

In 1972 the Board of Trustees of the American Hospital Association presented the following Patient's Bill of Rights with the expectation that observance of these rights will contribute to more effective patient care and greater satisfaction for the patient:

1. The patient has the right to considerate and respectful care.
2. The patient has the right to obtain from his physician complete, current information concerning his diagnosis, treatment, and prognosis in terms that he can understand. He has the right to know the names of the physician responsible for coordinating his care.
3. The patient has the right to receive from his physician information necessary to give informed consent prior to the start of any procedures and/or treatment, except in emergencies.
4. The patient has the right to refuse treatment to the extent permitted by law and to be informed of the medical consequences of his action.
5. The patient has the right to every consideration of his privacy concerning his own medical care program.
6. The patient has the right to expect that all communications and records pertaining to his care should be treated as confidential.
7. The patient has the right to expect that within its capacity an institution must make reasonable response to the request of the

patient for services.

8. The patient has the right to obtain information on any relationship of the institution to other health care and educational institutions insofar as his care is concerned.
9. The patient has the right to be advised if the institution proposes to engage in any research projects involving him.
10. The patient has the right to expect reasonable continuity of care.
11. The patient has the right to examine and receive an explanation of his bill regardless of the source of payment.
12. The patient has the right to know what rules and regulations apply to his conduct as a patient.

Furthermore, all activities of an institution must be conducted with an overriding concern for the patient and, above all, recognition of his dignity as a human being.

REFERENCES

1. Standards for Certification and Participation of Skilled Nursing Homes in Medicare. U.S. Department of Health, Education and Welfare, Sub Part K.
2. Developing Public Policies and Procedure for Long Term Care Institutions. American Hospital Association, 1975.
3. Classification of Health Care Institutions. American Hospital Association, 1968.
4. U.S. Department of Health, Education and Welfare, Public Health Service, Vital Statistics of the United States, 1944-66. U.S. Government Printing Office, Washington, D.C.
5. *Long Term Care,* by Samuel Levy and N. Paul Loomba, Vol.1. Spectrum Publications, Inc., New York, 1977.
6. Nursing Home Care in the United States, Failure in Public Policy. Special Committee Report on Aging, U.S. Senate, U.S. Government Printing Office, December, 1974.
7. *On Becoming an Aged Institutionalized Individual,* by M.A. Lieberman and M. Lakin. Atherton Press, New York, 1963.
8. United States Department of Health, Education and Welfare, Division of Program Operations and Procedure, May 19, 1971, pp. 1-2.
9. United States Department of Health, Education and Welfare, Social and Rehabilitation Service, Assistant Payments Administration, 1971, pp. 49-71.
10. United States Department of Health, Education and Welfare, Social and Rehabilitation Service, Aging, Administration on Aging, March-April 1972, p. 23.
11. *Hospital and Nursing Home Management,* by Robert P. Mathieu. W.B. Saunders

Co., Philadelphia, 1971.
12. Long Term Care Facility Improvement Study. National Center for Health Statistics, 1975.
13. *Nursing Home Fact Book*, 1970-71. American Nursing Home Association, Washington, D.C., 1971, pp. 5, 13.
14. *Nursing Home Administration: The Administrator's Role*, by Sidney D. Wallace. Futura Publishing Co., Mount Kisco, New York, 1974.
15. Nursing in the Skilled Nursing Home, by M.B. Miller. *American Journal of Nursing,* 66:325, 1966.

Chapter 4

ENVIRONMENTAL CONSIDERATIONS IN NURSING HOME PLANNING

INTRODUCTION

MANY diseases could be influenced through greater concern about the patient's environment — water, food, general sanitation, hygienic practices, nursing, and medical care. The task confronting administrators is the establishment of a framework for early detection of harmful environmental factors to reduce the chance of disability and premature death from disease. We must realize also that we cannot nicely distinguish the care needed by older patients with long-term illnesses from the care of a general medical nature. Integrated into the nursing home must be a plan to provide comprehensive care to all of its patients — a multitude of services to be called upon when needed. The first step in effecting any services is the periodic reevaluation of a patient's physical status, his psychosocial state, and the economic resources available. Knowledge of the history of the disease includes an understanding of the interaction of the cause, the host/patient, and environment encountered.

The facility is a combination of environments that interrelate to make up a whole. The goal of the facility is influenced by the interaction of the subsystems. The intent of an administrative body can be meaningless if proper attention is not given to all components of the system. In essence, an appropriate balance of environments and atmospheres must be maintained if the goals defined are to be achieved. Each component of the system is dependent upon the other.

The key to designing a nursing home for the aged is to focus on the needs, general requirements, and diseases of the population who will be using this facility.

The total environment includes the physical environment, the health care needs, and the service aspects of the facility. A concern for the proper environment of this facility in the area of atmospheres and attitudes will be most helpful in the planning of the proper setting for its overall purpose. Activities occur in spaces that are designed for them, but unfortunately the residents may not like the space or atmosphere allotted for an activity; thus, there is lost space and no proper setting for the activities.

Elements in an Interactive Facility

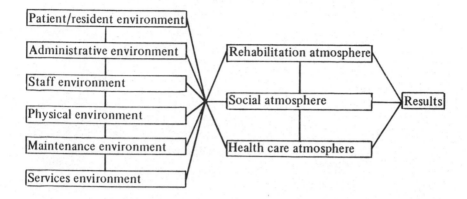

FALLING AND OTHER HAZARDS

Elderly patients, due to their handicaps and to their decreased physical strength, are more apt to fall than other people. Some hazards are uneven floor surfaces, highly polished floors, throw rugs, stairs, and objects in the way of free circulation. With proper planning, these hazards can be reduced. Floor surfaces can be non-skid types. Throw rugs can be removed. Wall-to-wall carpeting in some areas will help eliminate the hazard of falling. One of the most frequent times for falls is when the aged person gets up at night to go to the bathroom. Therefore, a simple, direct route from bed to bathroom will help patients. In addition, a light will help direct patients to their destination. Another element that causes falling is the decline in vision of the elderly patient; therefore, a nonglare light should be installed in the rooms, halls, and other areas.

Another common ailment related to age is loss of sense of smell. The elderly cannot detect gases that could be harmful. Automatic shutoffs, if gas supply has been interrupted, should be mandatory.

Bells and buzzers can serve as alarms. This brings up the subject of hearing, which in many people has declined, especially in high sound frequencies. All alarms should be on a low frequency and ring louder to enable the hard of hearing to get the message.

Another important element is temperature of the building and of the water. The hot water supply should never be above 100°F. because the elderly person can easily be burned at temperatures above this. Elderly people are very sensitive to drafts and inadequate heat. In the winter season the temperature should be 80° F. Large areas of glass should be curtained because they cause cold spots. The heating system should be controlled in each room to please the occupant's needs. In warm climates if ventilation is not adequate, elderly patients are subject to heat prostration and dehydration. Low or high humidity may also contribute to the discomfort of the patient/resident.

MOBILITY

How people move from place to place within the nursing home is of paramount importance. Most homes should be built with a wheelchair in mind, since many patients use them and need to be helped. Those that do not use them can benefit from the added space, making everyone more self-sufficient. Circulation depends upon the provision of adequate space for wheelchair use. Paths of circulation must be simple and direct with sufficient space to turn the wheelchair 180 degrees to clear furniture and other objects. Doors should be at least three feet wide to accommodate both the crutch cases and wheelchair cases. Thresholds should be eliminated between doors. The floor surface should be smooth. Ramps are needed for entry into the building.

The standard size of a wheelchair is as follows:

Length: 41½ inches
Width: 24 inches
Height: 3 feet overall
Height to arms of chair: 29 inches
Height, seat to floor: 19½ inches
A folded chair, width: 10 inches

Ramps

In any discussion on ramps, it must be pointed out that a steep sloping decline is a serious hazard. It is very difficult for patients to handle this by themselves because they can lose control going down, and going up is extremely tiring. The best suggestion is about one inch of slope for every three feet of the ramp. This is a workable ramp for the majority of elderly patients in a wheelchair. If the ramp is more than 15 feet long there should be a level area of 3 feet at the end of the fifteen feet for resting, then continue the ramp until the end. Furthermore, the ramp should be laid with nonskid surfaces with handrails about 29 to 32 inches high on both sides.

General Considerations

In all areas used by wheelchair patients, such as recreational rooms activity rooms, dining rooms, and lounges, a clearance of 30 inches is usual for the patient to get in under the surface of desks, tables, lavatories, counters, etc. The distance of a person's reach is another problem. This problem and others like it will determine the position of shelves, telephone, doorknobs, light switches, and electrical outlets.

PHYSICAL ENVIRONMENT

The first requirement is that the facility must have an open systematic design. The environment can be seen as paralleling the life functions and biological needs of humans. The physical plant is viewed as a separate entity containing mechanical systems to serve the real functions of the human organism. The word *facility* means the absence of difficulty. To call a building a health care facility indicates that the structure is allowing its functions to be accomplished.

The functions to be carried out by this facility are medical, social, administrative, and rehabilitative. A facility is the people and a physical setting acting in response to the people's needs. All of these elements, and each aspect of a nursing home, have their own environment. The physical environment must interact with other

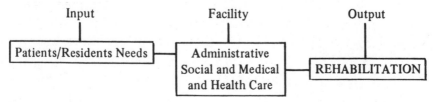

systems because each is a subsystem of a larger system. The preceeding diagram illustrates this point.

There are many basic environmenal areas, or atmospheres, that in most cases influence a patient/resident. In these areas the patient/resident will make his efforts to deal with the staff and personal needs. The patient attempts to maintain self-reliance and dignity and engage in living activities in this atmosphere.

Common Spaces

The typical spaces allotted in facilities for the aged are as follows:

1. Patient's/resident's room
2. Lounge
3. Corridors
4. Dining room or area
5. Entrance areas
6. Reading room
7. Bathrooms
8. Physical therapy and/or occupational therapy and/or general activities area.
9. Beauty parlors and barber shops
10. Worship services area or chapel

At the present time, the bulk of rooms are designed around the nursing staff. Yet, others who work in a facility that is so designed do not like it. The problem in many cases is that the residential design creates a great distance to service the patient, e.g. food services, laundry. There must be a balance of environments, which includes atmosphere and arrangement of areas, to achieve the goals of the facility.

If the occupant of a nursing home is designated as a patient/resident, then it follows that he is a patient because he receives health care and rehabilitation services. He is a resident because he lives there and should control space to the maximum degree possible. For every occupant the degree of control is different. The patient's/resident's rooms should be their sanctuary, yet the majority of nursing homes have two patients in a room. There should be only one patient to a room. The present arrangement of having roommates creates many problems to the detriment of the patient's/resident's well-being, namely, privacy and residential quality.

The private room should be adequate for socializing. How is it possible to have a homelike atmosphere with two in a room and no space to move except into the bed? The nursing home allots space for lounges, entry halls, and large dining areas. However, then the visitor goes past these areas and comes to the patient's/resident's room, he finds that the patient/resident is in bed; consequently, the visitor must stand or sit in the one chair available. The other occupant of the room shares the visit unless he leaves.

It is interesting to note that when a visitor comes to tour a facility, the tour is conducted in reverse order of access by the patient/resident. The visitor sees the exterior first, then is shown a nice large lounge, treatment rooms, activity rooms, dining room, corridors, nursing stations, chapel or area for worship, the offices of the administration, and finally the patient's room. Patients penetrate the same environment from the other direction. They reside in a room, go directly into a corridor, proceed to the lounge and then reach the dining room.

At this point in discussion of the environment, it should be noted that rehabilitation does not occur only in a physical therapy room or activity area or in an occupational room. It should be part of the overall planning of the facility. Rehabilitation occurs in every area of the facility. Many devices used in specially designated areas, such as ramps and rails, can be put in other areas for use all the time. Such devices could be put where access is natural and be made a part of the entire environment. This will encourage the staff of the nursing home to promote their aims and objectives at all times.

Nursing homes segregate people according to their mobility status. This makes it much more difficult for the staff to operate because of the heavier burden on the people who have to work at all times with less mobile types of patients. A mixture of types might be more interesting to work with than one type of patient. Although the therapist has classes of mobility within each of the categories, he will find people who do not particularly need a controlled environment; rather, they are seeking attention.

The typical bedroom found in a nursing home is a two-bed arrangement, with beds parallel. The orientation of the beds places one bed close to the window wall and the other near the closet and doorway. This arrangement usually means that the person in the bed next to the window feels "ownership" of the window, and the person located next to the door feels the same about the doorway and closet. This causes a subdivision of ownership because one person controls the lights and ventilation, while the other controls visitors, storage, ingress, and egress.

This room arrangement is very unsatisfactory, but it is common because of the cost of space. This hardly leaves room for a wheelchair around either of the beds. The space between walls and bed, furnishings and beds, fixtures and beds, and between beds is insufficient. The way the arrangements are made leads to damage to furnishings and possible injury to patients' hands, feet, legs, and arms due to contact with surfaces and edges while moving in wheelchairs and during transfer from them to the bed.

It is suggested that when bedrooms are being designed the entry door be in the center of the wall that faces the window. In rooms with two beds it would be possible to place the beds against the side walls, the foot of the beds facing the window, and the headboard against the wall. The benefit of this arrangement is that during nursing care, serving of meals, and other duties of the staff, it is easier to carry out the necessary functions upon entering the room. Many people have hobbies or activities that could be easily integrated with their programs of rehabilitation.

In order for a nursing home to have the feeling of being homelike, one must allow the patient/resident to have some control over his immediate surroundings. The lounges do not mean much to him because they are only used when entertaining visitors. This area is used by patients/residents with their visitors because these are the only places that visitors can sit and talk with some privacy. The patient's/resident's room is usually too small, and the other occupant of the room may be present.

Control over the physical environment by the patients/residents is all-important to their well-being. This control depends on five factors:

1. Mobility — The most common types of patients found in a nursing home fall into the following categories:
   a. Full ambulatory
   b. Disabled ambulatory (walks with crutch, cane, or walker)
   c. Semiambulatory (wheelchair bound)
   d. Nonambulatory (bedridden).
2. Personalization of room — The ability of the patient/resident to manipulate the physical objects within his room is important, in-

cluding the furniture, his personal effects, and any element that allows him to feel sympathetic towards his surroundings.

3. Socialization — The ability to mingle with fellow patient/residents both in public and in private areas without regulation or interference should be possible.
4. Privacy — There must be a place where every patient/resident can go, or retreat, that will permit seclusion for meditation, consultation, intimate discussion, personal activities, and rest. The most logical place for these activities is the patient's/resident's room.
5. Identification — The patient/resident must feel that he belongs in the facility. It is a two way street. The patient/resident and the nursing home interact, forming a single entity. This relationship will exist if the proper physical environment is present and if the administration and staff work along the same lines.

Through observation and discussions with patients/residents in nursing homes that provide both single and double occupancy, the patient/resident who has a private room is happier with fewer behavioral problems and fewer problems with the staff.

In general, putting two strangers in one room is very detrimental. In many cases, the staff will report that the coin-habitant of a two-bed room has contracted the physiological and psychological symptoms of the other occupant, even though there was no basis for these symptoms. One patient/resident may affect the health of another by proximity even though neither of the residents has a contagious disease. Seldom are two inhabitants of a room compatible. Generally speaking, this incompatibility is harmful to rehabilitation and to basic physiological and psychological health. It also violates all sense of privacy for the patient/resident.

The room must be designed to accommodate a high degree of personalization. Older people usually surround themselves with "clutter," which is representative of markers of a lifetime. To divest residents of these things is to take away very important clues about their ability to control their environment. This results in the patient's retaliation in some form: (1) changing behavior and (2) uncooperativeness. What better way is there to get back at an unsatisfactory environment? This gives the staff a new problem to work with and takes up more of the staff's time.

SURROUNDINGS

As important as the patient's room is his surroundings, which play a significant part in his life. Upon entering a nursing home, one notices the corridors, the lounges, and the residents sitting around, sleeping, and talking. Elderly patients wish to participate in or observe activities, which is why so many sit in the corridors. They will sit at the terminus of a hallway. There they can watch the activity over quite a distance. The same is true where hallways meet in the corner of a building. If you would make these areas attractive for the patients, then you will be giving them a place to meet. These corridors and hallways are ideal spots for lounges for the patients and places for activities and social behavior. Although the corridor is specified as an area of unencumbered passage, especially from the standpoint of safety and fire hazard, its attractiveness and relationship to the neighborhood make it a multifunctional space. To deny that social behavior takes place in the corridor and not to provide amenities for this to happen is to double the safety problem and make the hallway increasingly hazardous. If these spaces are not developed as suggested, patients will congregate there anyhow, bring things to use for their activities, and block the hallways.

The corridors must be considered transition space from the patient/resident room both in the social context and in the terms of traffic flow. The meeting and greeting going on in the corridor is important and should be facilitated by its design. A serious problem associated with a corridor is the inability of patient/resident to distinguish one area of the corridor from another or one corridor from another. The difficulty involved in institutions is the repetition of the elements in the corridors. Their similarity in the lighting system, low light levels, the glare of highly polished floors combined with excessive corridor length are elements that provide a very difficult environment to negotiate for people with sensory deprivation problems. The human sensory system is geared to perceive differences. In fact, where differences have been unconsciously designed out of an environment, the human sensory system will have difficulty perceiving location and place. There are ways of using these corridors for socialization. Marking off social areas, arranging chairs to break up space, or making the area different by easy perception of place and location are ways to make each corridor different. There should be variations on this theme throughout each corridor; thus each corridor would be more definable, and though the length is the same, they each would have their unique qualities and identities. Free passageways can also be expedited by careful designing of systems of interest. In fact, designers and planners should make every attempt to reinforce signals about location by various inserts. It is possible that visual, auditory, and textural inserts or clues can be carefully implanted to tell people where they are.

LOUNGES

The lounge area in most nursing homes is the result of regulations on the number of square feet that must be devoted to lounge space on the basis of the number of beds in a nursing home. This usually results in one or more very large areas devoted to socialization, relaxation, and contemplation. In reality, the space is seldom used for the purposes for which they were designed. In many cases the large space cannot be used for intimate conversation between two or three people. At other times this space is used for two or three different types of activities at the same time, resulting in confusion by participants. It is interesting to note that the arrangements of furnishings of the lounge are for ambulatory people to sit. Yet, in most nursing homes between 30 percent and 70 percent of the people in the lounges are in wheelchairs, and when visitors arrive they have to rearrange the furniture.

Lounges can either be isolated and enclosed with access through a doorway or passageway, or they can be open areas near an entrance. They can be at the intersection of hallways or in a space just off a corridor on one side or both sides. The isolated lounge may be less attractive than the open lounge because there is less potential for activity. One of the drawbacks to the open lounge is that so much is going on it interferes with discussions, intimate communications, and activities that need a degree of isolation to be effective. As lounges stand today, they are not, for the most part, fullfilling their intended role.

Lounges should be smaller and more accessible to the whole population within the nursing home, and this means transferring lounge space to patients/residents room space. The lounge in itself is a waste of space and money.

DINING ROOM

In the nursing home, there is one activity that is by far the most popular — eating. Going to the dining room does offer an opportunity for a patient to divest the mind of thoughts about sickness and decreasing lack of capability and to think and talk about something external to problems of self. Dining rooms in most nursing homes are utilized only about 50 percent of the time. There are two reasons for this:

1. A substantial proportion of the patients cannot go the the dining room; they must be provided with means in their rooms.
2. A number of patients will not go to the dining room because of their embarrassment over appearance, their inability to eat without help, or the condition of the space itself.

For many of the patients, dining rooms can be very noisy, resulting in conversation becoming indistinguishable from the background noise.

The dining room itself is designed for seating as many people as possible without consideration of the patients. There is a special need for passageways between tables, for space to serve the food and to get wheelchairs under the table tops. Many of the chairs in the dining room have arms that do not allow them to be pushed close to the table.

Another problem that arises with the use of a dining room is the number of patients that are to sit at a table and the shape of the table, i.e. round, square, or rectangular. The round table is more accessible because the supports are in the middle and not on the corners.

A thoughtfully planned, pleasant dining room will mean that more of the patients will use it. It can serve the dual purpose of feeding the patients and of providing an area for socialization. Those using chairs with arms and those using wheelchairs should be able to get in close under the tables. Ingress and engress into the dining room and from the tables after eating should be planned so that the patient has sufficient space for mobility.

A nursing home environment is just as important as any other element of rehabilitation. The patient/resident will be aware of this and will feel at home, which, in turn, permits a greater opportunity for rehabilitation.

ENVIRONMENTAL STRESS

It has been suggested that environmental stress may accelerate the aging process, and when occurring in old age, it is important in the production of psychiatric disturbances. The traditional milestones in old age that must be passed successfully are (1) retirement, (2) bereavement, (3) rejection, and (4) isolation.

Retirement

Basically, there are two reactions to retirement:

1. It has been described as a public disrobing ceremony in which the victim faces the prospects of reduced income, no occupation, and excommunication from the company of his business friends. Perhaps the individual who finds retirement an obstacle is one whose resources are already strained to the limit, one who has never made plans for the future, one who has no inner resources, has no hobbies, and has seldom been able to cope.
2. To many it is an opportunity to a fuller life. These are stable people who have always been able to cope and who have enjoyed all stages of life. Retirement to them is simply the next adventure.

There is little real evidence that retirement per se plays a part in the production of mental illness in the elderly. In fact, women are less likely than men to be affected by retirement, and yet mental illness is more prevalent in elderly women than men.

Bereavement

It has been shown that bereavement is a significant factor in mortality rate. Married men who have lost their wives show an increased mortality rate for the first six months following bereavement.

Isolation

There are two main groups of social deprivation:

1. Lack of material things — income and housing
2. Lack of family and/or friends

There is evidence to show that these factors are related to mental illness. Social interaction is a necessity for maintenance of mental alertness.

Rejection

All those who work with the elderly are familiar with the feeling of rejection that their patients experience. The behavioral disorders of psychiatric illness are more prone to produce rejection of the victim by relatives and family than severe physical disabilities are. One is often confronted with this problem in nursing homes where the family and relatives are unwilling to accept the patient back into their home in view of past experiences. They fail to tell the patient that it is not possible for them to provide adequately for them, which inevitably results in a deterioration in morale and physical well-being.

The extent of organic brain damage may be due to the degree of environmental stress. The human organism requires time to adapt to change. If it has been slow in onset, organic change and environmental stress, even of a severe degree, are much better tolerated and produce less impact.

The facilities available to patients who have mental problems are limited. There is the constant problem of whether these people belong in a separate facility for mental disorders or whether they should go to a nursing home that takes all types of patients. Which is the better equipped to handle mental patients? It is important to the nursing home that they be prepared to take proper care of all types of patients.

The type of environment that they give these patients will play an important role in their recovery. The planning is all-important. The elements that go into the environment are the size of the home, the number and types of patients, the orientation of the patient and employees in the handling of patients, and the ability to treat these patients as people with problems who need their help.

THE INFLUENCE OF THE ENVIRONMENT ON PATIENT CARE

The structure of a nursing home may implement or impede the type of performance of patient care received in a nursing home. Deep consideration must be given to the elements of the building design in order to insure the development of interpersonal relationships and smooth operations of rehabilitation and other types of programs.

Basic Requirements

1. Landscaped entry with good outside lights. A nice entrance in the rear is also helpful.
2. Weather conditioning for both heat and air, with individual room controls in bedrooms for heat and cool.
3. Soundproofing of ceilings and walls. This type of installation will permit the patient more privacy by keeping out noise.
4. Separate circuits and silent switches throughout the building.
5. In case of fire, a sprinkler system and an alarm loud enough for all to hear are essential.
6. Ramps in place of stairs. There are many ambulatory, semiambulatory (in walkers), and wheelchair patients who will curtail their activities rather than brave steps.
7. Flush mounted light fixtures to prevent glare and the collection of dust.
8. The window should be pivoted and open outward. Shatterproof glass should be used. If windows turn outward, there is less likelihood that patients will hurt themselves on an open window.
9. Doors should be recessed in the walls with push-pull handles and roller latches to keep them closed.
10. Separate plumbing circuits for plumbing and toilet facilities so that an entire area does not have to shut down in case of trouble.
11. Mat-operated opening of front doors in entrance to the building. These can be operated by an electric eye.
12. Kitchen, dining areas, and recreation areas conveniently located close to patients' rooms.
13. Built-in furniture to allow more space for patients.
14. No raised thresholds.
15. Alarms on all exterior doors, which would be activated at night, so that if a patient wanders off, there would be an immediate warning at the nurses station.
16. The use of wall paint that can be seen easily by the older person.

Accessories to the Environment

1. Large clocks and calenders in plain view of patients.

2. Footboards and safety belts in all beds to be used if necessary.
3. A book shelf-desk combination built in bedrooms with the desk height set to accommodate a wheelchair.
4. Bed lamps that are adequate for reading in bed.
5. Storage space for out-of-season clothes.
6. Lockable drawers to help prevent articles from being stolen.
7. Bulletin boards where they can be seen.
8. A daily newspaper.
9. All clothing of patients should be clearly marked, preferably by the family.

Special Facilities

1. Beauty care and barber facilities.
2. A dining room-recreation room combination may be a way to save space.
3. A garden and court area.
4. A physical therapy area.
5. A room for special projects and general use — speech therapy, crafts, meeting room, etc.
6. A lounge and/or lobby.
7. Emergency equipment room.
8. A library and music room that could be used for recitals, conferences, meetings, group therapy.
9. A staff lounge.
10. Public toilets in lobby.

REFERENCES

1. *Designing the Nursing Home,* by Joseph A. Koncelik. Dowden, Hutchinson and Ross, Inc., Stroudsburg, Pennsylvania, 1976.
2. *Planning Homes for the Aged,* by Geneva Mathissen and Edward H. Noakes. F.W. Dodge Corp., New York, 1968.
3. Environmental Factors in Dependency, by Tom Arie. In *Care of the Elderly,* edited by A.N. Exton-Smith and J. Grimley Evans. Grune & Stratton Publishers, New York, 1977.
4. Environments of Geriatric Care. In *Clinical Geriatrics,* by Isadore Rossman. J.B. Lippincott Co., Philadelphia, 1971.
5. Environmental Setting and the Aging Process, by Robert W. Klemier. In *Psychological Aspects of Aging,* edited by John E. Anderson. American

Psychological Association, Inc., Washington, D.S., 1956.

6. *Housing for Aging,* by Wilma Donahue. University of Michigan Press, Ann Arbor, Michigan, 1954.
7. American Standards Association, Making Buildings and Facilities Accessible to the Physically Handicapped, American Standards Documents, A. 177,1, 1961.
8. Facilities for the Aging, by Clinton H. Cowgill. *Journal of American Institute of Architects,* Part 1, May, 1960.
9. *Rehabilitation Center Planning,* by Cuthbert Salmon and Christin F. Salmon. An Architectural Guide, University Park, Pennsylvania, 1959.

Chapter 5

TYPES OF DISABILITIES FOUND
IN NURSING HOMES

TYPICAL REACTION TO DISABLITY

A LIST of typical patient reactions to disability due to various psychological factors follows:

1. The exaggerated and overdetermined response to disability
2. The predilection for disability
3. The use of denial of disability
4. Hopelessness and helplessness reaction
5. Expression of anger at incapacitation

In the first instance, the treatment must take the problems into account and develop a treatment plan with them in mind. The treatment must include —

1. an awareness of the exaggeration of the patient's response;
2. recognition of the major determining factors;
3. distinguishing the sensitizing factors in the past from the present real situation;
4. resolving the past conflicts contributing to the overdetermined present response.

In cases of denial, some patients refuse to believe that there is any hope of getting well. In other cases, they refuse to accept disability and express confidence that they will eventually be completely well. The staff handling cases of denial may experience frustration and anger. This response is because the patients' denials contradicts the staff's ideas and pronouncements. These patients are frustrating because their attitudes imply that any results other than complete recovery will fall short of the goals subconsciously set by the denial and, thus, of the expected results. The staff should not become angry. If they do, the patients will respond by resisting their attempts to help. If the staff supports the patient's denial, it will affect the patient's cooperation in the rehabilitative program. The best way to treat this individual is not to contradict or confirm the denial but to give strong support to his more adaptive behavior.

Patients who show anger will often display (1) irritability, (2) fault finding, and (3) outbursts at people around them. Usually the supportive personnel and the team specialists get the brunt of this anger. This makes for a very difficult situation.

The reaction of patients is very important, but so is the reaction of the personnel who work with these patients. It must be realized that the long-term care of nursing home patients, the severity of the disability, the unique social situation, and the complexity of individuals all contribute to the development of intense personal relationships between patients and the staff.

There is a variety of staff reactions to a patient who manifests the denial of disability by anger and rejection. The patient's overt hostility or aggressive behavior has been discussed. There are three other types of staff-patient reactions that need to be studied and understood: (1) mutual hopelessness, (2) staff helpfulness, and (3) sex.

Mutual Hopelessness

Each patient has different degrees and different stages in which they feel more hopeless at certain times than others. The staff's reactions to the periods or moods have a great deal of influence on the patient. The staff act as a temperature gauge for the patients and reflect the patient's moods. The staff, if they are eager, want improvement. In some long-term cases, this eagerness acts as a pep pill to the staff. If they do not get the results, however, they start to give less and less attention to the patient. Naturally the patient senses this change and responds slowly to the rehabilitative program. In a sense, both the patient and the staff started out overenthusiastic. The patient was overoptimistic, and the staff encouraged this belief. Consequently, if the patient was making slow progress, this was not enough. Therefore, it is important to remember never to be overly optimistic. One should stay within the bounds of reality. This will enable the staff members and the patient to work toward the long-range goals at a speed that will produce the best results. Hope must be tempered by reality. Slow progress is the most realistic and important characteristic of rehabilitation goals for the elderly. Measurements and evaluation will keep the patient and staff within the bounds of reality.

Staff Helplessness

To watch patients fall and to stand by and just give advice about how the patients can pick themselves up is one of the hardest tasks to teach the staff who work with long-term disability patients. Most patients want to become as independent as possible, particularly in self-care, or everyday living activities. All people trained to work with patients who have disabilities are encouraged to help them help themselves. The staff members usually go into the field of rehabilitation because they feel the need to help. In the early stages of a patient's disability, helping him is very important. Soon, the patient reaches another stage in convalescence. In this second stage, continuing to help the patient to the same degree as in the first stage is defeating the rehabilitation process. Suddenly it is not right for the staff to help patients sit up. They can do so with the trapeze bar that they have been learning to use. The staff members must watch them struggle to succeed. It is much easier to give them help and not stand by, and it takes twice as long to see if they can succeed on their own.

Too much help from the staff can actually impede the patient's progress toward self-care. This process is a difficult and painful one for both the patient and the staff working with them. Patients with disabilities of long duration must learn responsibility for their own functioning.

Patients are able to manipulate their staff workers. Many of them learn how to approach the staff on their weaknessess and, thus, appeal in a way that cannot be refused. They get therapists to do things for them that they could do if they were not lazy.

Members of a staff must recognize each other's weaknesses and help each other. If the nurse tells the physical therapist that a certain patient is not feeling well and will not attend the physical therapy period, then it is up to the physical therapist to see the patient to ascertain whether the patient is indeed ill. This must be done in such a way not to hurt the nurse's feelings. Talk the patient into realizing the need for going to therapy and act as the buffer between the nurse and the patient. Gain patients' support; they need to go because they will feel better after the therapy. Convey this to the nurse, who should have realized that the patient took advantage of his good nature.

CARE AND TREATMENT OF THE CHRONICALLY ILL

A large percentage of every nursing home's population is labeled chronically ill. This is because must persons over the age of 55 years have some disorder or some malfunction of their circulations, their bowels, their bones and joints, or their nervous systems.

There are many factors outside of disease that make a person chronically ill:

1. Mental unfitness, the lack of a disciplined mind, loss of curiosity, or drive
2. Physical unfitness, the lack of using the body properly
3. Social deprivation, lack of family or friends
4. Occupational unfitness, lack of a job resulting in a loss of financial independence
5. Nutritional unfitness, poor diet plus poor eating habits

One must remember that a chronic disease cannot be cured. In rehabilitation there is hope. Rehabilitation goes beyond the physical and psychological; it must include social situations and other related areas if it is to be effective. The primary concern is the participation of the patient if there is to be any measure of success. Many patients who are labeled chronically ill have a rheumatic disease.

All older people show some evidence of a musculoskeletal deterioration. Some have rheumatoid or degenerative arthritis, gout, or difficulties associated with a stroke or a fracture. To the extent that function of the musculoskeletal structure is impaired, the individual is deprived of participation in the sociophysical activity of life around him.

Teamwork of all members of a rehabilitation team is the only hope for the maintenance of optimal function of the patient who is chronically ill. In many cases, the key person, the patient, is the least effective member of the team. One of the major objectives of the members of the team is to work in a manner that will include the patient. The key factors for being successful is a proper prognosis.

As soon as the physician has made a diagnosis, the team begins to educate the patient to understand the reality of his illness. He needs to understand that a single drug or a single activity will not cure his illness or rehabilitate him. It must be pointed out that a complete cure may not be possible, but prevention of crippling deformity and improvement of function is possible, which presents the greatest hope for all concerned. This, of course, includes the prevention of development of patient's mental attitudes that will inhibit the use of his limited musculoskeletal system.

Understanding mental reactions, training the physical activities, orienting the staff, instituting drug therapy, and providing proper diet are elements of successful rehabilitation.

CHRONIC ILLNESS AS A PROBLEM IN ADAPTATION TO LIFE

When a person is chronically ill, it becomes a permanent factor in his life. Ill health is of necessity seen from a psychological point of view. Ordinarily, acute disease represents a rather abrupt change in an individual's life and is accompanied by increased stress, tension, and frustration due to altered function. We know very little about the psychological effect of disease when it is persistent for months and years. We are not able to sort out readily and to differentiate alterations in behavior due to the long-term altered function or to the regular pattern of the individual.

It is very important to understand that people who finally become aware that they have a chronic illness must be studied and techniques developed for evaluating the capacity of the patient to make adaptations in the face of prolonged ill health and the resultant disability.

In order to understand which would result in helping patients, we need to study the following areas: (1) motivation, (2) level of aspirations, and (3) tolerance for frustration.

In the case of the chronically ill person, one must realize that the individual has very definite emotional drives as a result of being chronically ill. This may help both the patient and those involved in his care to direct the energy of emotional drives toward a wholesome and reasonable adjustment to the illness. It may also aid the patient and the staff to understand the various steps in the direction of the drive toward a healthy mental and emotional balance or to appreciate the steps that may turn the direction of the patient's emtional drives toward increasing anxiety and insecurity with resulting difficulty.

Among one's individual emotional drives and needs the

following are found:

1. An urge toward aggressive dominance
2. A longing for submissive security
3. A need for the satisfaction of good health
4. A desire to love and be loved
5. A drive to obtain an opportunity for self-realization

It may greatly help both the chronically ill patients and those who are helping them to evaluate the relative pressures of these emotional factors in each case. With the onset of chronic illness, a patient naturally feels emotional disturbance, anxiety, and insecurity.

The first step in orienting the psychodynamic forces in an individual toward a satisfying personal and social adjustment is to help him obtain self-knowledge, a growing understanding of self and environment. With increasing self-knowledge and understanding, the patient might be aided in an effort toward a balanced satisfaction of the emotional drives and needs that are involved. These can be reached in the face of the circumstances of the particular chronic illness, and the environmental conditions present.

It is equally important for the patient with chronic illness and all those who may be involved in the care of that person to realize the various steps that may go in the opposite direction and to recognize them as promptly as possible in order to try to turn the drive toward the positive healthy balance. The first sign seen among patients is the development of symptoms of anxiety and insecurity. These result from the diffuse unconscious fear that the basic emotional needs of the individual may not be satisfied. The continued force of the lack of basic needs of the individual would tend to operate from anxiety to insecurity and then to frustration. There may be great emotional disturbance in the sick person, and those who are involved in the care of that person may become distressed at the apparent failure of their efforts.

A characteristic feature of frustration seems to be the tendency to focus the unpleasant and hostile emotional reaction on some individual close to the frustrated person. This may be the physician, the nurse, a relative, or anyone else with who the frustrated person comes in close contact. The focusing of frustration may follow a pathway of acute symptoms leading to resentment in which the diffuse emotional feeling of frustration becomes sharply pinpointed on a specific person who is then considered responsible for the emotional distress that the frustrated person may feel. In normal health one can get rid of frustration in various ways, such as active participation in sports or merely watching them. However, there is more of a chance in chronic illness of focusing frustration than in ordinary life. The chronically ill do not have many opportunities for explosive relief; thus, there is more of a chance to focus their frustrations on whatever is at hand.

This situation points out the need and importance of early training in the promotion of directing the emotional needs of an individual toward self-knowledge, self-understanding, and realization. An active effort toward the balanced satisfactions of emotional drives and needs would result in mental health and emotional security and equilibrium. It is of the utmost importance to do everything possible to direct chronically ill people toward an active search for satisfaction of their emotional drives and needs.

People with chronic illness do have many complicating psychological problems relating to themselves, friends, and the staff workers in the institution. Those who care for the chronically ill patients also have psychological problems. A clinical psychologist should work within the framework of the rehabilitation team. Full coordinated teamwork can aid in getting the facts for planning and carrying out the program.

PHYSICAL DISABILITIES

Certain physical disabilities occur more frequently in the elderly than in any other age groups for which there is a great need for rehabilitation. The most common disabilities are caused by musculoskeletal and neuromuscular disorders, cardiovascular diseases and metabolic diseases, pulmonary problems, and cancer. As a result —

1. 50 percent need help in ambulation;
2. 25 percent cannot ambulate at all;
3. 67 percent are chronically ill;
4. 33 percent are convalescent.

Fractures of the Hip

Since one of the most frequent fractures that occur in elderly people is the hip fracture, injury will be given more attention than fractures of other areas. In many cases, during the forced period of convalescence required to recover from hip fractures, the patient develops secondary disabilities that can cause more harm to the overall recovery of this patient than the original fracture. The most common types of immobilization are the following:

1. Impacted fracture is a condition in which the fragments are severely compressed. This calls for conservation treatment, which includes bed rest and proper positioning.
2. Internal fixation, in which a pin is forced through the trochanter and the femoral neck into the femoral head.
3. Prosthetic replacement.

Some ways to manage hip fractures are as follows:

1. If the fragments are impacted and held together, it is best to do nothing.
2. Internal friction of the hip is carried out by forcing a nail through the trochanter and the femoral neck into the femoral head.
3. Remove the fractured portion of the femoral head and neck and replace them with a metal femoral head using a long stem into the medullary canal of the femur.

It usually requires about three weeks for healing of a surgical wound. During this period, all strain should be avoided to prevent stress on the sutures and to prevent slipping of the prosthesis.

Rehabilitation

With impacted fractures weight bearing must wait until the bone is healed. This takes about three months. The patient will have restricted mobility, and when allowed up, he should use crutches for ambulation at first. Isometric exercises should be given to maintain general strength.

In internal friction procedures, the patient is in bed only during the period for the surgery to heal, usually three to five weeks. Then he is allowed to learn to ambulate.

The complete replacement of the hip joint has become the most popular method of repairing hip fractures. More details about the rehabilitation follow:

BED PHASE. This may be from one day to one week, depending on the patient's condition.

BACK LYING. The prosthetic hip and knee are flexed to 15 degrees. The leg is rotated medially and maintained with a sandbag or towel roll under the trochanter. The bed is flat or the upper portion could be rolled up to 15 degrees.

SIDELYING. This is done on fractured side only. In no case should the patient be allowed to lie on the uninvolved hip. No exercises are done at this time with involved hip. Bed exercises are allowed after the first week if the physician orders them (depending on the patient's condition). If allowed, patients can try turning themselves and can try to use the trapeze to exercise the arms, trunk, and shoulders. The feet can be exercised if a brace is not on the leg. If the patient is not in pain, he can be placed in a chair with leg positioned in medial rotation. Start with one hour and increase slowly.

STAND–UP POSITION. This is permitted after patients have gained strength in chair with no pain. It is easier for patients to try to stand from chairs that have the seat elevated a few inches than from normal chairs. They can put most of the weight on the uninvolved leg and gradually put more weight on the involved side, depending on pain and tolerance of patients. They should do range-of-motion exercise, while standing, at least ten repetitions of each motion three times a day.

Other Fractures

FRACTURE OF THE SHAFT OF THE FEMUR. Short fractures are less common in the elderly patient. In these cases, skillful nursing care is very essential, as the extremity is put into traction. As soon as the fracture has shown some clinical firmness and early healing, a single plaster hip spica splint is applied, and turning and mobilization are begun. It is possible to teach walking with some weight bearing in such a splint.

FRACTURE OF THE TIBIA. A walking cast is used for immobilization, which allows early walking with partial weight bearing using crutches or a walker for support.

FRACTURE OF THE ANKLE AND FOOT. The use of a cast is necessary for the ankle. The same applies to fractures of the tarsal and metatarsal bones of the foot.

FRACTURES OF THE CLAVICLE. The figure-of-8 bandage is used to keep the shoulders back and elevated and to immobilize the clavicular articulations with the sternum and the scapula.

FRACTURE OF THE HUMERAL NECK. A sling is used for one to two weeks, then pendulum exercises are started.

FRACTURE OF THE HUMERAL SHAFT. The rule in humeral shaft fractures is conservative treatment, for example, the use of a hanging cast for upper humeral fractures, which provides weight for traction when the sling is properly applied.

FRACTURE OF THE WRIST. Wrist fractures are very numerous in the elderly population. Colles' fracture is the most common. They are usually immobilized in a plaster cast. Early treatment is absolutely necessary to preserve function of the fingers.

VERTEBRAL FRACTURES. This happens in elderly patients who have osteoporosis, which predisposes compression of vertebral bodies. It may also be caused by trauma. Usually the patient must remain in bed for about a week to allow the very painful period to pass. Then the patient is fitted with a back support, and ambulation is started.

DISLOCATIONS

Dislocations are treated the same as fractures, by reduction and immobilization. The immobilization period must be long enough for the joint capsule, ligaments, and other soft tissues to heal before any movement is allowed in the affected areas.

SPINAL CORD INJURIES

There are a variety of causes of spinal cord damages: falling on the head, athletic injuries, car accidents, fights with knives or guns, etc. If the spinal cord in injured, function is lost or impaired in areas at and below the side of the injury. Loss is both motor and sensory. The degree of impairment is directly proportional to the extent of the spinal cord injury and typically produces motor and sensory paralysis or weakness, loss of reflexes, loss of bowel and bladder control, and disorders of generative functions.

The result of a lower cervical spinal cord injury will be quadriplegia involving all four extremities and the trunk. In paraplegia, the lesion is in the thoracic or lumbar region, and only the lower extremities and trunk below the lesion are involved. In hemiplegia, the lesion is on one side of the brain with injury of varying degrees to cortical cells, which originate in the brain and receive impulses from descending or ascending spinal cord traits.

Early in patients' rehabilitation, nursing service is by far the main source of help to these patients. They can prevent secondary disabilities such as bed sores and contractures. The quadriplegic whose injury is in the cervical spine will always require some care in the management of his body and of his life. Care for the paraplegic depends on the level and extent of the spinal cord injury. The paraplegic with a high thoracic lesion has no involvement of the upper extremities. Usually he can get in and out of a wheelchair and is fairly independent in his everyday living activities. In some cases, full bracing of the lower extremities is possible, but primarily they are confined to wheelchairs. The patient with a midthoracic injury has good upper extremities and thoracic stabilization. On level surfaces, the patient can ambulate with braces. The paraplegic with low thoracic lesion has, in addition, some abdominal muscle strength. With braces, he can climb stairs and curbs. The patient with low lumbar or sacral injury requires limited bracing and is completely independent in all activities, with only moderate deficiencies in ambulation and in some elevation activities.

Hemiplegia

The term hemiplegia refers to a paralysis of the muscles of one side of the body which results from damage to parts of the brain on the side opposite the muscular impairment. The brain areas usually affected in the hemiplegia are the cerebral cortex, the brain stem and the pyramidal tracts.

This injury is usually caused by a cerebrovascular accident (CVA), an arterial hemorrhage, or obstruction. Obstruction may be caused by a thrombosis when a blood clot forms locally in an artery or by an embolism when loosened blood clots or an air bubble travels in the bloodstream and lodges in a cerebral artery, causing blockage, or occlusion, or collapse (spasm) of a cerebral artery. Hemorrhage follows a rupture of a blood vessel. Thrombosis and hemorrhage are usually found in the artereoscleratic vessels, hence, in older people. If hemorrhage is the cause of CVA, the blood that has escaped from the vessel enters brain tissue and forms an expanding lesion with increased pressure and symptoms.

Regardless of the cause, the result of a CVA is a failure of circulation of oxygen carrying blood to an area of the brain. The consequences of this is damage or death of the brain cells of the involved area. Ambulation and the use of the upper extremity of the affected side are prevented or restricted. Hemiplegia may involve corticobulbar as well as corticospinal tracts; hence, there will be, in addition to the paralysis or paresis of arm and leg, contralateral lower facial paresis. Often, hemisensory loss is present. If there is brain damage in the dominant cerebral hemispheres, on the left side if the patient is right-handed and vice versa, it results in language damage. This will be discussed under aphasia.

Aphasia

Aphasia refers to the loss of language such as speaking, writing, telling time, reading, typing, counting, recognizing things, and understanding communications. There are three general types of aphasia:

1. Expressive Aphasia: The inability to express oneself primarily through the medium of verbal and written communication. It is a disorder of the language output. Expressive aphasics will experience difficulty in finding words, naming objects, using words in proper order, counting, telling time, typing, spelling and writing. Often they do not make sense in speech and do not realize it.
2. Receptive Aphasia: A disorder of language input. It is the inability to understand either spoken or written language. Such patients become confused when given instructions and when reading, since these activities require correct reception by the patient. If a patient has equal difficulty in both using and understanding language, then they have mixed aphasia.
3. Global Aphasia: The complete loss of all language skills.

Speech Disorders

Speech disorders occur in hemiplegia patients. The common term for this affliction is dysarthria. It is an organic disorder in speech production resulting from impairment of the speech musculature, such as incoordination, paralysis, or weakness. It produces impairment of respiration, phonation, articulation, volume, rate, and voice quality. The most common dysarthric speech symptoms are slurred, disarticulated verbal production.

VERBAL APRAXIA. Verbal apraxia is the inability to perform purposeful movements of the speech musculature. There is an inability to move the tongue, lips, and appropriate facial muscles voluntarily.

Brain Damage

Brain damage is defined as a wound or injury inflicted, usually suddenly, by some physical agent. The term brain damage is not a very useful one to describe people's problems because it does not describe the extent and the location of this damage. Certain injuries will produce spastic paralysis. A patient might have an upper motor neuron injury that will cause the loss of voluntary movements. Injuries that occur above the muscle's point of origin (supranuclear) give rise to hemiplegia or quadriplegia. If the injury occurs in the midbrain or below, there is specific cranial nerve involvement or paralysis of cranial nerves on one side of the body. It is important in rehabilitation to know the exact location of the lesion in order to know why a patient responds certain ways and has limitations.

Encephalitis

Encephalitis is an infection of the brain that may be localized or diffused throughout the brain tissue. It may be an extension of meningitis, which is an inflammation of the membranes that surround the brain and spinal cord. Patients that recover from this disease may have the following signs or symptoms: They will have neurological, intellectual, and emotional impairments. Signs or symptoms are some paralysis, blindness, aphasia, deafness, and cranial nerve defects.

Parkinson's Disease

Parkinson's disease has slow progression of lesions of the pyramidal or extrapyramidal system. Usually found in the elderly, it is caused by arteriosclerosis. Characteristics are the following:

1. Increasing ridigity of muscle tone.
2. Slowness and difficulty in initiating and executing voluntary movements.
3. Tremor.
4. Tremors are likely to be more severe during relaxing than during voluntary movements.
5. Alternating flexions of the fingers produce the pill-rolling tremor.
6. The facial lines are smooth and expression fixed.
7. Tongue muscles usually are involved.
8. Speech becomes slurred and soft.
9. Posture is usually stooped with the head down.
10. Gait will be short, slow, shuffling steps, with hands by side.
11. Patients will stop in middle of stride, called freezing.

MUSCULAR AND MUSCULOSKELETAL DISORDER

Back Pain

Back pain is usually caused by trauma, excessive effort, strain, or stress. Strain of any of the muscles or groups of muscles that attach to the spine will produce damage to the muscle or its tendon, producing local hemorrhage that may result in some scar tissue. The elasticity of the remaining muscles are reduced temporarily by protective spasm. In many cases, poor postural positions will cause trauma to develop in elderly patients. Conservative treatment is usually successful. If not, then one must look for a reason why the person is not getting well.

Arthritis

Arthritis is the inflammation of a joint.

Osteoarthritis

In the process of aging, there are certain degenerative changes that take place in articular structures. If there are articular tissue changes, which grow to more than normal proportions, these produce major defects in the articular surfaces. This results in mechanical friction and irritation with consequent inflammation and pain as the irregular articular surfaces move against each other. The joint inflammation or arthritis is a result of friction upon use of a joint, produced by intra-articular changes. The most common affected parts of the body are usually the weight-bearing joints and those joints most subject to trauma, such as knees, hips, and lumbar and cervical vertebrae. Just as often the terminal interphalangeal joints of the fingers and the carpal-metacarpal joints of the thumb are affected.

Rheumatoid Arthritis

Rheumatoid arthritis is the most frequent and most disabling arthritis. Once a person contracts the disease he has it for life. Interestingly enough, there is no one factor or combination of factors that has been established as the cause of the disease.

Symptoms are as follows:

Specific — Pain, swelling, stiffness, wasting of muscles, limitation of range of motion, deformity, in degrees

General — Fatigue, insomnia, depression, agitation, anorexia with weight loss, fever, chills, anemia

In general, there is no prediction as to the growth and development of this disease. It can develop rapidly and in one year can cause death or grow by slow stages over the years.

Heart Disease

Heart disease is one of the biggest health problems; it causes about 1 million deaths per year. The patient with heart disease is one person who really needs understanding and rehabilitation. There are several types of heart diseases, but they all have some common symptoms:

1. Heart failure, caused by the heart pump not functioning correct-

ly. If the pump fails to function properly, there is a feeling of weakness or fatigue. The patient tires easily doing activities that did not bother him before.

2. Chest pains. Pain is in the center of the chest below the sternum. In many cases, the pain is not very severe and goes away quickly. In setting up the proper rehabilitation program for heart disease patients, one must classify according to their activities. This classification is done as follows:

Class 1: Have no limitations in physical activity. Their normal activities do not produce any symptoms of heart disease.

Class 2: Have slight limitations in activity and are comfortable at rest. Ordinary activity results in fatigue and palpitation.

Class 3: Have marked limitation of physical activity and are most comfortable while resting. Any slight effort will bring symptoms.

Class 4: Have discomfort doing any type of activity. These people need to be in bed or in an armchair or wheelchair.

Amputations

It is interesting to note that 75 percent of all amputations are carried out on people over the age of sixty years. Amputations are done on all extremities usually due to some pathology that can only be arrested or cured by taking off some part of an extremity. In most cases, it is the lower extremity. Some causes that might be mentioned are vascular deficiency (usually due to diabetes), tumors, accidents, and infections. Let us briefly examine the questions as to the types of amputation.

1. Hemipelvectomy — half the sacrum and the entire hip bone is removed. Prosthesis is fitted, but the patient always has an awkward gait, but he can ambulate successfully.
2. Above the knee.
3. Below the knee.

In all cases of amputation, a prosthesis, properly fitted and followed by rehabilitation, will enable patients to carry out their normal functions. One of the problems is the elderly patient who can use a prosthesis but refuses to try to use it. The key to rehabilitation with a prosthesis is that the patient desires to have one and then has motivation to succeed in using it. Use of a prothesis varies with the with the patient's needs. It is best to classify amputees according to anticipated functional activities when considering a prosthesis:

Class 1: Full restoration. These are expected to be fully functional, they can do most anything they have done before.

Class 2: Partial restoration. Can do most anything, but not as long nor as well. May have to limit their activities.

Class 3. Very limited function. Can do their own everyday living activities. Their needs vary from patient to patient. They cannot ambulate well alone and cannot use steps without help. Another group here can do some of their daily living activities but cannot carry them out alone.

Osteoporosis

A patient with osteoporosis usually complains of low back pain. This is a condition whereby bone mass becomes reduced while the bone itself remains identical to normal bone. This is written up on elderly patients as senile osteoporosis. There are many factors that cause this disease, but the one most important cause comes from the lack of activity usually due to a fracture, causing osteoporatic changes in the immobilized areas. Some of the symptoms are back pain, in various degrees but usually in the sacral area. To help this patient, one must get them active and out of bed.

Gait Patterns

Gait patterns is a classification that is added to give the rehabilitation team a better idea of what causes elderly patients to ambulate as they do. As a result of poor gaits, patients develop pathological problems that interfere with their ambulation. Motor ability in the elderly is generally considered poorer in aged persons. There is a gradual decline in accuracy and speed in motor performance, which is due to physiological aging and brain damage. Another reason why people have poor gaits is because they were bedridden for a long time due to other causes. Proper rehabilitation will enable this patient to become normal again. Poor gait may be due to arthritic changes, which may occur in hip or knee, causing a change in gait because of pain. Another cause could be the length of time the patient was forced to stay in a wheelchair. Certain names associated with gait patterns might help in understanding them:

Petren's Gait: This gait is a result of neurological impairment. Most cases resemble the gait of a person who has Parkinson's disease, with sole, dragging, short steps.

Double Step Gait: Patients with hemiplegia, hip fractures, and locomotor disorders exhibit this type of gait. Usually the patient takes two steps and stops to regain his balance.

In closing this discussion of gait patterns, it should be mentioned that some other causes of changes in gait patterns are (1) disuse, (2) pain or changes in the alignment of the bones of the legs, (3) hip fractures never healed, (4) nerve involvements, (5) motor system diseases, (6) spinal cord diseases. Rehabilitation is the only hope for these patients. More details will follow in other chapters on gait and gait training.

NERVOUS SYSTEM

Following is a brief explanation of the nervous system. The brain is divided into specific areas which control different organs and different functions of the body. It activates, coordinates, inhibits, and controls functions as well as stores information for future use. It is a superb computer when all its elements are intact.

The neuromuscular apparatus that controls voluntary motion, mobility, and locomotion is a combination of several areas in the cerebral cortex, which are connected by many association neurons.

The upper motor neurons that initiate voluntary motion arise in the cortices of the right and left cerebral hemispheres. After being modified by association with neurons from other areas, they descend, cross to the opposite side just before entering the spinal cord, and finally make contact with lower motor neurons in the gray matter of the cord, which innervates all voluntary muscles of the limbs and trunk. Muscles of the head are innervated by cranial nerves, most of which are also crossed. Also crossed are the muscles of speech, which are controlled by an area adjacent to the lower part of the motor cortex. The premotor area, which exerts a great deal of control by way of association fibers, is separated from and anterior to, the motor cortices. The topographical sensory area lies just posterior to the motor cortex and is separated from it by the central sulcus.

The neuromuscular areas have two basic divisions:

1. The sensory component, which carries impulses to cells in the brain, originates peripherally, and makes many connections within the brain.
2. The frontal association centers are important in mental activities, such as learning, memory, attitudes, behavior, etc. The parietal association centers are necessary for the correlation of cutaneous sensations. The occipital lobe is the visual center; the temporal lobe is related to learning.

Thus, neurological impairment can cause the following:

1. Impairment of thinking and intellectual functioning, e.g. mental retardation, collectively known as the "brain syndrome." Brain syndrome is a comprehensive term for mental disabilities.
2. Impairment of motor function
   a. Loss of muscular strength, paralysis, or weakness, lower motor neuron lesions
   b. Loss of muscular control spastic paralysis, upper motor neuron lesions
   c. Loss of coordination and equilibrium, e.g. cerebellar ataxia
3. Sensory impairment — blindness, hearing loss, loss of skin sensation, loss of proprioception, etc.

MENTAL DISABILITIES

Brain syndrome is associated with the following characteristics:

1. Decrease or defects in orientation
2. Memory loss
3. Decrease in the patient's fund of general information
4. Decrease in the patient's ability to do simple calculation.

Brain syndrome also refers to losses or defects that are psychiatric reflections of organic brain damage manifested by the aforementioned symptoms, all of which can be hidden unless one carefully looks for them.

Brain syndrome is caused by loss of brain cells, which comes from —

1. severe head injuries;
2. infectious diseases with high fever, such as encephalitis, meningitis, and scarlet fever;
3. deficiencies in nutrition which may act as an agent for loss of brain cells;
4. genetic inheritance;
5. senile deterioration.

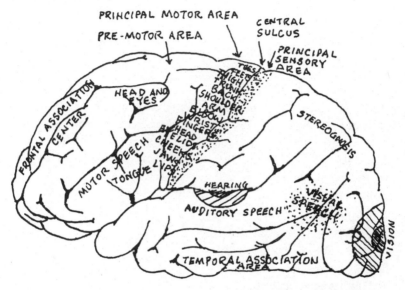

Figure 5-1. Cortical projection and association areas on the lateral aspect of the cerebrum.

TESTING PROCEDURES FOR BRAIN SYNDROME

Use both tests listed below.

Mental Status Questionnare

Questions	*Answers (indicate awareness of):*
1. Where are we now?	Place
2. Where is this place (location)?	Place
3. What is today's date and day of	

day of week?	Time
4. What month is it?	Time
5. What year is it?	Time
6. How old are you?	Memory
7. When is your birthday?	Memory
8. In what year were you born?	Memory
9. Who is president of the U.S.?	Memory
10. Who was the president before him?	Memory

Face-Hand Test

Examiner and patient sit down facing each other. The patient is asked to put his hands on his knees and his feet flat on the ground and to close his eyes. The examiner simultaneously touches the patient's cheek and hand, and the patient reports, by word or sign, where the touches were. The test procedure is one of double-simultaneous stimulation, usually in this order:

1. Right cheek, left hand
2. Left cheek, right hand
3. Right cheek, right hand
4. Left cheek, left hand
5. Right cheek, left cheek
6. Right hand, left hand
7. Right cheek, left hand
8. Left cheek, right hand
9. Right cheek, right hand
10. Left cheek, left hand

If the patient makes errors, the examiner tells him to open his eyes and then repeats the test. In most cases, there is little or no improvement in the retest. It has been found that similar scores on the two tests are almost always measurements of organic brain syndrome.

A patient may become confused when given simple instructions such as sit down, hands on knees, close eyes, wait until examiner touches you, report to the examiner where the touches are. In many cases, after all these instructions are given a patient will get angry and refuse to go on or he will not be able to remember. This proves the patient is untestable due to brain damage, because he cannot grasp the subjects or understand what he is being asked to do.

PERSONALITY AND BRAIN SYNDROME

What is a personality? Is it how a person reacts to his environment, or is it how a person reacts to other people in the nursing home?

People have different behaviors for different occasions. Can we find any direct connection between brain damage, emotions, and behavior? What are signs of brain damage? Is it intellectual deficit? What about people's moods? Do changes in mood of aged people reflect brain damage?

Many aged people are irritable. One of the signs of old age seems to be the inability to tolerate frustration. One sign that is seen most often in nursing homes is depression. Much of the personality change that is thought to be a consequence of aging and brain damage may actually be a reflection of the individual's response to aging and his limitations and also his attempts to deal with these.

The question in staff workers' minds in dealing with aged people in the nursing home as related to their behavior are as follows:

1. Is the patient acting in this manner because he has brain damage, and is frustrated because he cannot do things that he formerly did?
2. Is the patient acting up because he feels that he could do better if he gets the help he needs from the staff members of a rehabilitation team?
3. Is the patient acting up because he has brain damage that has affected him mentally and because he does not understand? If this is the situation the only treatment is medication.

Changes in personality could simply be the same person adapting his behavior to a new and different situation. The degree of mental and physical impairment must be determined to ascertain the amount of damage that has occurred to the brain.

If the assessment of degree of impairment is accurate and the areas of impairment can be specified one is less likely to push patients with brain damage to emotional overreaction.

Also, one must not dismiss as organic, and therefore irremedial, the disturbed and seemingly confused behavior of an older person, which, in fact, is symptomatic of depression. The prognosis for depression is good if the patient is given proper care and treatment. With aging of the brain, learning capacity may remain just as good but may take longer. Multiple stimuli may lead to perceptual failure and decrease pleasure. An older person may enjoy music more with his eyes closed and no one on stage than when sight and sound are simultaneously stimulated. People are complex and unique.

EMOTIONAL DISORDERS AND BEHAVIORAL PROBLEMS

The patient who says "I am lost without you," or "I can't walk down the hall by myself," or "Who will take care of me when you go off duty?" are overly dependent people. Usually they are scared because of decline in health and can do less for themselves; thus, they become more dependent and frightened. They have in the past always needed the approval of people. It could be that some staff workers need to have people depend upon them for their own self-esteem. This is dangerous. Workers in a nursing home should realize that their purpose is to encourage independence in the patient.

Another type of patient that is prevalent in the nursing home presents a behavioral problem that must be understood. This is the formerly independent person who finds that due to declining years he has developed both physical and mental weaknesses and who tries to hide it from the staff and from his family. Upon entry into a nursing home, this patient is depressed and uncertain for the first time — a new experience that frightens him. The patient needs to discuss the situation with someone who can help him understand it.

In many cases, physical rehabilitation will improve the patient, and through other phases of rehabilitation mental and social attitudes can be improved. The nursing home staff must remember that it must not put such a demand on a person's physical and mental strength that they cannot achieve success in the home. There must be provisions to compensate for any physical or mental defects that a person has sustained.

INDIVIDUAL BEHAVIOR AND SPECIAL PROBLEMS

Fighting among patients and temper flare-ups present another problem. Many actions in the community are not noticed, but due to the closeness and the lack of privacy, actions of patients in a nursing home are judged very harshly. Patients discuss other patients who have lost their tempers. They realize this is dangerous behavior for all the residents of a nursing home. The fight may be caused by a patient who wants attention or one who is angry; however, the age and the physical state of the participants make for a real danger.

People in the nursing home have been put there to be taken care of. Therefore, they expect the staff to protect them from themselves and from others in the home. In some cases, patients develop problems due to a brain syndrome about which they have no knowledge. Thus, they react now to situations that in the past were just minor irritations.

The reasons patients withdraw from society are numerous:

1. They feel superior and thus do not want to mix with the others because they do not know how.
2. Perhaps they are not capable of doing what is asked of them either by staff or fellow patients; thus they withdraw to hide their inabilities. They also may not be interested.

In handling these situations, the staff needs to study the backgrounds of all patients and discuss them at great length to come up with a proper solution for each situation that occurs. The patient of a nursing home is in a confined group situation. Many of these people did what they wanted in public and were never compelled to hold their tempers or to behave themselves. Anger, hurt, and frustration are some factors that need to be considered.

The staff must not accept as fact the first story of other patients. If they were not actually present when a problem arose, they must be calm about getting the facts. They must not make hasty decisions about who is, or who is not, the guilty party. Protection now and for the future depends on the staff's actions. The staff has the dual responsibility of getting the true facts and then of making decisions on how to handle these patients in the future. The patients must have the feeling that someone cares, that someone will protect them.

Sexual problems are another major concern of the nursing home. Many of these problems are due to lack of privacy. The other patients are watching, judging, and coming to conclusions that may or may not be true. The nursing home is not a wide open world. It is a close, intimate group that makes its own standards for its society. Any actions by the patients that might be approved in the outside world may be censored, forbidden, and condemned by the residents of a nursing home. Furthermore, what may be acceptable in one nursing home may not be acceptable in another. This is due to locale, the people involved, and the ways the administration makes its decisions on these issues.

In many chronic handicaps, such as quadriplegia, the disabilities will affect sexual function from a purely physical standpoint. Everyone knows that a sexual life is important to adjustment. The staff must contend with the following problems: Is the patient wondering what is happening to his spouse? Does the patient get sexually aroused? For the rehabilitation of the patient physically, mentally, and emotionally, isn't this a factor to be considered? What can be done must be done by the rehabilitation staff. Some inquiry should be part of the staff evaluation before and during the rehabilitation process to identify potential major complications to the patient's recovery. For example, the staff may be concentrating on teaching a patient ways to become independent and stronger while his major concern is that his wife was considering divorcing him because she feels that they never will have normal sexual relations again. It is true that in some handicaps patients will never recover adequately to function as they did before the illness or accident. Therefore, the staff must try to get patients and their spouses to discuss this and work out a satisfactory solution to the problem. Adjustment and understanding in the area of sex must be recognized by the staff members if they are to help the handicapped person become rehabilitated.

In the brain-damaged or brain syndrome patients we have been discussing, one must remember that many of these people are not capable of being rational. They are not capable of logical discussion. They are brain damaged. In many cases, they are easily led into actions by people who are more dominating and who thus get their own ways. The brain damaged are not cognizant of their responsibilities and obligations to others, nor are they aware of their social responsibilities to others. The question arises, Do you have time to worry with the patients' behavioral problems? Many nursing homes say it takes their staff all day to just keep their patients/residents clean, fed, and well protected.

THE DEPRESSED PATIENT

Depression is an affective disorder — one kind of mood disorder. The term depression can be applied to disorders that appear to be genetically determined or programmed into the person and which occur periodically. Such recurrent disorders may be called mood cyclic disorders. The cycle may be recurrently depressive, recurrently manic, or alternating. Mood cyclic disorder is probably more common than is generally believed. Also, depressive reactions can have multiple and interrelated causes. Depression, whatever its type, is very common in old age. Understanding of depression is often facilitated by recognition of the following signs:

1. Resignation to a defect — either physical, such as the loss of a leg, or mental, such as the wandering mind.
2. Hopelessness.
3. Anger — at self or at others, sometimes called rage. People who commit suicide are usually angry at themselves for getting into an unacceptable situation. Also, they may be angry at a situation they cannot solve. Others are demanding people, always wanting something, or they are complainers.

Society has told people that at a certain age they are old. As a result they are supposed to accept certain aches, pains, and disabilities. Resignation, hopelessness, anger, suicide, rejection of reality, and demanding and complaining, especially to family and the nursing service, are not the answers. Should one ignore these signs or do something about the conditions that bring on the depression?

SYMPTOMS OF DEPRESSION

Symptoms of depression include the following:
1. Insomnia in the early morning, waking up during the night
2. Anorexia, poor appetite

3. Changes in bowel movements, constipation or diarrhea
4. Decline in energy, listlessness, fatigue, inertia, psychomotor retardation
5. Loss of interest in usual pursuit
6. A lowering of spirits, feeling blue, sad, and down usually in the morning, and feeling better as the day goes on
7. A longing for bed, early retirement, and quickness to sleep
8. Somatic complaints, fears, expressions of guilt, worthlessness, or loneliness
9. Paranoid trends, irritability, vengefulness, spite

These are the signs to look for to help understand patients and to give them the best possible care. It is not likely that the staff members will give them treatment, but symptoms should not be ignored. They should be brought to the attention of the physician, by making notes in the patient's chart and trying to discuss them with the physician.

The main point that the staff worker needs to remember is that these signs or symptoms are patients' searches for relief from their sufferings. Furthermore, if the staff recognize these symptoms and relates to the patient, they can be supportive and reassuring to the patient and help decrease feelings of helplessness. This is the type of support the patient is seeking. Giving time by listening and discussing his problem is evidence that staff members consider him a worthwhile investment.

The depressed person/patient must recognize that staff members are trying to help, that they are involved. Inaction drives the patient to continue this inefficient, unconstructive pattern of behavior.

In many cases, physical decline and depression may coexist. Illness and infirmity may have more than a casual relationship to depressed feelings. The loss of resources for adequate functioning leads to feelings of helplessness. Depression, in turn, aggravates illness and impairment.

As a result of the study of the patient/resident, the staff may find that there are some things that can be done to diminish stress:

1. Diminished hearing can be helped by a hearing aide.
2. Dentistry can relieve pain, improve patient's appearance, and increase the number and kinds of foods the person can eat.
3. Prostate problems may need surgery.

4. Hemorrhoids can be treated.
5. Uterine prolapse can be corrected.

These are examples of health problems common among old people. Improvement in health is accompanied by an easing of the depression and by improved emotional health.

Envy of others is common with depression. Depressed people envy others because they do not seem to be depressed and suffering. They avoid healthy persons and start withdrawing from the group. Depressed people must be watched carefully. Their environment must be studied. They need a protective and supportive environment in order to feel reassured.

These people need an uncomplicated facility, which maximizes their ability to learn their way about from their room to the dining room, to the lavatory or toilet, to the shop, to the recreation room, and to other areas of activities. They need staff workers with time, patience, and skill to help them in many ways. They need supportive persons, who see to it that they eat, bathe, go to the toilet, keep themselves clean, and go to bed.

Some nursing homes put all patients together regardless of physical or mental problems. Others segregate the mental cases from the physically disabled. This is better in most cases; however, segregation should depend on the patients concerned.

Depression is the most common of the functional psychological disorders in older persons and can vary in duration and degree. It may be precipitated by loss of a loved one or the onset of a physical disease.

The psychologic characteristics are the following:

1. Irritability
2. Indecisiveness
3. Feelings of hopelessness
4. Confusion
5. Dissatisfaction with self
6. Devaluated self-image
7. Thoughts about suicide

Staff members should watch for these psychologic warning signs as well as the physiological signs listed previously so that depression can be caught and treated as early as possible.

MULTIPLE DISEASE

Unlike young people, the elderly frequently suffer from multiple diseases and ailments. Elderly people bear the permanent defects of past injuries, illnesses, and operations. They accumulate diseases that can be controlled but not cured, such as pernicious anemia and myxedema, diseases that disable but do not kill, such as osteoarthritis, osteoporosis, and cataracts, and diseases that are potentially lethal but chronic diseases, such as atherosclerosis or diabetes. The frequency of many diseases rises with age, such as malignancies, stroke, depression. Parkinson's disease and fractures are a few examples. New diseases arise against a background of preexisting disabilities and also from a slow decline in the functional capacity of most bodily systems, resulting from physiological or nonpathological age changes. Thus, respiratory reserve, renal function, and many homeostatic mechanisms such as temperature regulation and the control of blood pressure and posture all show steady decline with age.

Multiple diseases and disabilities may summate and interact so that a number of minor lesions that would be of little consequence individually may be important together. Thus, heart failure may often be due to the combined effects of several trivial pathologies. For similar reasons, complications of the primary illness are far more likely in the aged.

The elderly person complains of pain less often. Conditions that are usually accompanied by severe pain in the young may be totally painless in old age. Many heart attacks come with a minimum of pain. Many osteoporotic elderly have collapsed vertebrae but have no corresponding history of back pain.

The relative infrequency of pain in the elderly can be contributed in part to their greater stoicism, and pain may be more readily forgotten where there is mental impairment. Even when pain is experienced, elderly patients often find themselves unable to describe it accurately. Some elderly patients are the exception and complain long and loud of pains all over the body. Such multiple complaints of pain should strongly suggest the possibility of symptoms of a depressed patient. Changes in the severity or character of chronic pain should get special attention. It is all too easy to disregard such changes and so overlook a definite injury.

The symptoms of illness in the elderly are often misleading and different from that of earlier years. Many illnesses are present in an entirely nonspecific way or by mental changes. Some elderly are prone to minimize their symptoms; they are too ready to accept them as being their expected lot. They also are particularly likely to fail to call for medical attention promptly.

Illness in old age often is presented as an insidious and progressive deterioration, which may comprise a decline in social competence, appetite, initiative, and drive, together with growing frailty, loss of weight, and an increased likelihood of other illnesses. There is often some overlap with psychiatric symptoms such as apathy, deteriorating memory, and mental confusion.

Many chronically ill patients have physical handicaps that could be remedied by the use of rehabilitative personnel for treatment on a day-to-day basis. Some homes ignore mental problems of patients if they do not interfere with the routine of the home. Some illnesses are ignored because at the current rate the patients are paying they could not afford to furnish patients with the care needed for their ailments. Everyone agrees there is a need for services that would help all patients mentally and physically, but at the present time, it cannot be done due to the high cost of professional personnel. It is interesting to note that as a result of the admission policy set up, the administrator, and the director of nursing, patients that were classified as mental cases and were not allowed to visit their homes except on special conditions made adjustments that were satisfactory to the administration, i.e. these patients became withdrawn, apathetic, and uncomplaining.

Often administration is unwilling to get a psychiatrist to come in and study a patient unless the nursing home is unable to handle him. Too often they do not try to correct the patient's gradual loss of contact with reality, since the patient was not a behavioral problem.

The patient going from the hospital to the nursing home has problems. Perhaps the most critical point for the transition of the patient to the nursing home is in the first month after placement. Two factors enter into a successful changeover. The first is the patient's attitude towards the home. If he takes it in his stride and does not become anxious, angry, demanding, depressed, or withdrawn, then his chances for success are good. The other factor is the effectiveness of the administrator, the director of nursing and the nursing staff in dealing with the patient's problems. If the nursing staff through its director makes the patient feel at home and acts positively when the patient gets upset but does not itself overreact in an anxious manner, this maximizes the adjustment of the patient. Should the staff wait too long before responding to the disturbed behavior or before setting limits to certain behaviors, patients will go downhill fast and regress to the point where they cannot be handled. A balance must be struck between tolerance for uncontrollable behavior and firm management of behavioral disturbances.

Many patients entering a nursing home show signs of some impairment as demonstrated by symptoms of confusion, disorientation, and memory loss. Others show signs of auditory and visual impairments. Many cannot carry on the necessary activities of daily living. The treatment and care of these patients are influenced by acceptance or rejection of these behaviors by nursing home administrators and staff.

The abnormal behaviors that were most important in the nonacceptance of patients into the nursing home were the following:

1. Depressed patients. These were the withdrawn, retiring, and complaining people. Some were apathetic; some lacked interest in people and activities; some were slow in movement, speech, and thought; some had physical complaints.
2. Passively uncooperative patients. These were quiet, sullen, and stubborn, refused to follow routine, wandered off, got lost. Many got angry and refused to eat.
3. Disturbed, aggressive patients. These people threatened patients, destroyed property, were overactive, restless, and unpredictable in behavior, were very uncooperative, loud and boisterous in speech.
4. Agitated patients. These patients were confused, disoriented, and suffered from intellectual impairment. They usually could not do any of their everyday living activities. They usually were crying or laughing.

Many administrators would not accept these patients. They were too much of a burden on the staff of a nursing home, which did not feel qualified to handle them. If they were accepted, at the first sign that they could not be handled, they would be sent to a hospital.

Where could they go? Some administrators would take a few, but only for economic reasons. Administrators and nursing directors would take the physically handicapped patient rather than the mentally disturbed patient. When these patients are taken in, it is only because the physician in charge of the patient has agreed to be available on a twenty-four-hour schedule to treat this patient. In the majority of cases, a physician sees patients in nursing homes on an average of twice a month. Some administrators will take mental patients if they can get a psychiatrist to take care of a patient whenever he is called.

This is a common sense approach showing an interest in people. The nurse-patient relationship is perhaps the most important to the patient of a nursing home. The patient is dependent on the nurse not only for routine nursing care but also for satisfaction of such needs as socialization, information, and security against feelings of being lost and abandoned. The nurse should be on a first-name basis with the patient, should inform the patient of plans for treatment, and should encourage the patient to socialize with others, and to participate in social activities. The nurse needs to encourage the patients to hope that they can get well and provide reassurance that help will be given.

Another reason that patients become emotionally disturbed is because either the family or the physician did not tell them what to expect when they arrived at the nursing home; therefore, they are unprepared for this new change in surroundings. The director of nursing or the administrator must see to it that patients are immediately oriented to their new home. Patients who make an adjustment to the nursing home are the ones who are prepared for the new environment. These patients also have good relationships with other patients. Adjusted patients make friends with their roommates. They also find other patients with whom they are able to socialize. They are seen frequently by their physician, giving them assurance that they will be looked after.

REFERENCES

1. National Institute of Mental Health, Section on Mental Health of the Aging, Division of Special Mental Health Program, by Alvin I. Goldfarb, 5600 Fisher's Lane, Rockville, Maryland.

2. *Care of the Long-Term Patient*, Vol. 2, by the Commission on Chronic Illness. Harvard University Press, Cambridge, Massachusetts, 1956.
3. *Common Diseases in the Elderly*, by H.M. Hodkinson. Blackwell Scientific Publications, Oxford, London, England, 1976.
4. *Medical and Psychological Teamwork in the Care of the Chronically Ill*, edited by Molly Harrower. Charles C Thomas, Publisher, Springfield, Illinios, 1954.
5. *Medical Care and Rehabilitation of the Aged and Chronically Ill*, 3rd edition, by Charles A. Bonner. Little, Brown & Co., Boston, Massachusetts, 1964.
6. *Psychosocial Intervention Programs within the Institutional Setting*, by Leonard Gottesman and Elaine Brody. Edited by Sylvia Sherwood. S.P. Brooks, Division of Spectrum Publications, New York, 1975.
7. Neurological Disorders of the Elderly, by Simon Locke. In *Clinical Aspects of Aging*, edited by William Reichel. Williams & Wilkins, Baltimore, Maryland, 1978.
8. Rehabilitation of the Geriatric Patient, by Jerome Tobis. In *Clinical Geriatrics*, by Isadore Rossman. J.B. Lippincott Co., Philadelphia, 1971.

Chapter 6

INTRODUCTION TO REHABILITATION

INTRODUCTION

OUR society has changed from ignoring to helping the handicapped. This is evident in the voluntary organizations supported by contributions and to local, state, and federal governmental aid to the disabled.

Rehabilitation must be based on understanding the patient and knowing what goals are to be accomplished. Since rehabilitation is primarily concerned with human values, the whole person, his uniqueness, and his environment, the restoration of the disabled to a life that is purposeful and satisfying is the ultimate goal — providing persons who are disabled or impaired by reason of accident or illness, with an opportunity to function adequately as family members, citizens, and economic contributors. Rehabilitation can only be accomplished by a worker who considers each patient to be an individual. Every person has the right to participate in all aspects of life. Rehabilitation is not only a philosophy but a way of life — adjustment of a disabled person to his environment, his society, and his disability. Individuals should develop their intellectual, social, and vocational potential to the highest level possible.

Technique depends on the worker. Not every person can recover physically, mentally, socially, or economically to the level they were operating at before their disability. The patient and the people working with him must keep this in mind and continuously change their techniques as a result of new evaluations and progress of the patient.

To maintain the health of a patient over a long time, constant worker alertness on the patients' rehabilitation is necessary. Success will prevent or delay deterioration and will provide positive stimulation to the individual to improve his capacities and to maintain the highest level of independence.

As part of the technique, the staff members must recognize at an early stage of relationship between them and their patients that social and psychological adjustments go hand in hand with physical adjustments. As a result of an illness, personality problems that were hidden or controlled before the illness may arise. They may increase to the point of becoming a major obstacle to satisfactory adjustment. If patients have mental depression, they will not endeavor to improve from a physical standpoint.

Another important consideration in working with the patients are their families. In some cases, patients in a nursing home can be rehabilitated to a point that they can return to their own homes and communities. This active attitude looks for obstacles that limit functioning, induces the patient to recognize them, and then tries to motivate the patient to improve those deficiencies in and about him. It builds a moat that enables him to leave the prison of obstacles. It is a continuing effort to restore function and to reintegrate patient with family and community. At the moment, the nursing home or convalescent center is their home. The people in it are their families. The staff members are the people who can relate individuals to their needs.

Most patients need comprehensive care to restore lost or limited functional capacity for coping with the environment. This includes prevention of further functional deterioration from the effects of an existing disability. The team, which includes the staff workers who are in constant contact with the patient, must be aware of the needs of the patient and the individual program for each one. Alertness, patience, and compassion are mandatory for the success of a rehabilitation program.

The ultimate goal of the rehabilitation program is to return each patient to full function. However, this is idealistic because it may not be physically possible for each patient to regain full function. Thus, all concerned must realize that the return to full function is an ideal to work toward, but that it is a goal not possible for all patients. The realistic result will be when the patient attains his maximum amount of function and can make no further progress. Goals should be established in relation to the patient and in relation to the needs of the community. The goals of an institution provide a basis for its policies. For example, the institution's goals for rehabilitation of its patients will influence the types of rehabilitation services offered and the policies determined for its services.

It is important to remember that the fundamental idea in all rehabilitation is that a person is a total being — that he is composed of physical, mental, and social attitudes, which taken together constitute a whole person.

Rehabilitation is the process of helping patients use what movement and muscular energy they have remaining to obtain their maximum functional status. If they have loss of strength in one lower extremity, this would be the ability to ambulate with their residual muscular power. Braces, splints, prosthesis, canes, and crutches may be used. If they cannot ambulate, they must learn to use a wheelchair. If they have loss of function of the upper extremity, this curtails their activities of self-care and loss of independence in their daily functioning activities. Therefore, there is a need for retraining. They need activities for muscles of the arm, orthotic devices, muscle substitution, and self-help aids to restore a variety of functions.

FAILURES IN REHABILITATION

Failures in rehabilitation can be caused by the following:

1. patients' reliance on others to perform their necessary functions.
2. severe depression, mental confusion, and poor motivation.
3. lack of rehabilitation facilities or personnel.
4. excess dependency on family or friends.

HISTORY OF REHABILITATION

The history of rehabilitation is tied to the development of medicine. Throughout history, the handicapped have been ridiculed, persecuted, or ignored. Primitive people abandoned the disabled. Today, in many cases we segregate them. Hippocrates in his book on surgery described many deformities and said, "Keep in mind that exercise strengthens and inactivity wastes." This is still one of the basic principles of rehabilitation.

Early in history, various treatments were described. One was heliotherapy, use of the sun as a healing power. People worshipped the sun as god for its powers. Artificial limbs were recorded at the time of Hippocrates. The first known crutch was recorded on an Egyptian tomb. In 2380 BC Greek gymnasts taught massage. Then came the Dark Ages when the handicapped were again treated poorly.

In the fourteenth century, gunpowder was invented, and for the first time people were hurt and maimed by gunshot wounds, which had to be treated. This started rehabilitation, and each subsequent war stimulated more interest in it.

In the eighteenth century, British physician John Hunter described what has become the basis of muscle reeducation, namely, the relationship between the will of the patient and range of motion. By the end of the century, Philippe Pinel liberated the insane by beginning psychiatric rehabilitation. This was the first time that occupational and recreational therapy were used as methods of treatment. Physical and psychological care had begun.

In the late nineteenth century and the beginning of the twentieth century, major steps were laid for modern rehabilitation. The first interest was in treating crippled children. The use of idle time was called occupational therapy. During this time, medical social service was started. Home care was added to nursing education. The first visiting nursing service was begun by Lillian Wald. The first professorship of physical therapy in the United States was held by R. Tait McKenzie at the University of Pennsylvania in 1911. Then came World War I, which stimulated the use of rehabilitation. In 1919, the first issue of the *Archives of Physical Medicine and Rehabilitation* was published; it is now the official journal of the American Congress of Rehabilitation Medicine. In 1921, the first issue of the *Physical Therapy Journal* was published. In 1941, Doctor Frank H. Krusen wrote the first textbook on treatment methods called *Physical Medicine*. World War II brought Colonel Howard A. Rusk. He was able to demonstrate how rehabilitation would and could improve the lives of mankind. Since World War II there has been great growth and development in rehabilitation.

Today, even with increased knowledge, better education, and expansion of facilities and financial support, it is estimated there are still hundreds of thousands of persons who are being deprived of adequate rehabilitative programs. This is due in part to an inertia of both professionals and communities. Since a major objective is to add quality of life to any person who has a chronic illness or disability regardless of age, it is most encouraging that some health workers are accomplishing results once considered impossible. Rehabilitation services should be available to all. Without the benefits of a good program, many people are living at a level lower than their capabilities.

DEFINITIONS OF REHABILITATION

Rehabilitation means the restoration of the individual to the fullest physical, mental, social, vocational, and economic capacity of which he is capable. Doctor Frank H. Krusen (1972) says the following:

> Rehabilitation is a creative procedure which includes the cooperative efforts of various medical specialists and their associates in other health fields to improve the mental, physical, social and vocational aptitudes of persons who are handicapped, with the objective of preserving their ability to live happily and productively on the same level and with the same opportunities as their neighbors.

The Community Health Service of San Francisco (1960) defines rehabilitation in the following way:

> Rehabilitation is the process of decreasing dependence of the handicapped or disabled person by developing them to the greatest extent possible in the abilities needed for adequate functioning in his individual situation.

Helen J. Yesner, a social worker from the same service, defines it as follows:

> A treatment process designed to help physically handicapped individuals to make maximal use of residual capacities and to enable them to obtain optimal satisfaction and usefulness in terms of themselves, their families and their communities.

Other definitions of rehabilitation are the following:

1. Rehabilitation involves the treatment and the training of patients so that they may attain their maximum potential for normal living, physically, psychologically, and socially.
2. The restoration, through personal health services, of handicapped people to the fullest physical, mental, social, and economic life of which they are capable.
3. Rehabilitation is a creative procedure that includes the cooperative efforts of various medical specialists and their associates in other health fields to improve the physical, social, and mental attitudes of people who are handicapped. The objective is to perserve their ability to live happily.

Rehabilitation is a transient episode during which a human being with a physical or psychological impairment is given the opportunity to realize in himself latent potentialities for improved independence of action and of personal care. It stresses the qualities and determination of the patient to get well, and the physical arrangements come as a secondary consideration. Rehabilitation can seldom be carried out in a hospital room, no matter how talented the staff. Group interaction with other patients, the proper atmosphere, and a dedicated group of individuals on a twenty-four-hour day are essential for a successful rehabilitation program. In rehabilitation, one is dealing with a whole person with physical, psychological, educational, vocational, and social needs. Rehabilitation is not convalescence. It is the active participation of all the staff with the patients to restore them to their fullest capacity.

In the word rehabilitation, the root *habil* in Latin means able; thus, the simplest way of explaining rehabilitation is "making able again."

The aim of rehabilitation is not only to improve physical ability but to attempt to improve function within the limits and activities judged reasonable, to maintain without undue stress, and to slow down physical deterioration. In the area of physical defects, the goal is the prevention of secondary complications such as muscle contractures, ulcers, superimposed infections, and atrophy of muscles. The goals of rehabilitation must be realistic. The staff's energies should be directed towards offering the greatest potential for independence and improvement. The first target should be the area that bothers the patient most.

The person most involved and most important in rehabilitation is the patient himself. The patient needs the professional to show him the way, but if he is determined not to get well, then the professional cannot achieve the set goals. A patient can achieve some degree of success physically and in the area of independence by improving self-care activities, but to achieve the ultimate goals, one must have wholehearted cooperation motivated by a desire to achieve success.

UNDERSTANDING SOME TERMS USED IN REHABILITATION

The work *impairment* is frequently used. Tests and measurements reveal that a person has a disability, but it has not been determined how this impairment will affect a person. The word *handicap* is simply an extra burden that the individual must overcome to avoid a reduction of a specific functional activity. The word *disability* does not refer to an anatomical defect; it is used to describe the condition of a patient who cannot perform certain activities in a normal manner.

Also, it does not mean that a person is unwell. It could be said that an *impairment* could produce a *handicap,* which may result in a *disability*. Thus, by definition, an elderly patient is a handicapped person, since most aged people have some impairment that leads to a handicap, resulting in a disability. Because of this, social and recreational goals are altered, and spiritual values take on a greater meaning.

THE REHABILITATION TEAM

The usual members of the rehabilitation team are the physician, rehabilitative nurse, physical therapist, occupational therapist, speech therapist, social worker, recreational therapist, and psychologist or psychiatrist. In most cases, the nursing home will have the physician, a nurse, and, in some cases, a part-time consultant in the other specialties.

The question arises, Are all these specialists needed full time on the staff of a nursing home? The answer is no. What good is it for the speech therapist to work with a patient for one hour a day and for the remainder of the day to allow him to continue as before the lesson? The same principle applies to all the remaining specialists of the rehabilitation team. If specialists do work with some patients, staff of the nursing home must work together with them.

It is the author's contention that the key people of the rehabilitation team are the people who are in constant contact with the patients. They are the unsung heroes of any successful rehabilitation program. The LVN or LPN and the aides and volunteers are the workers. They supply the basic needs to the patient and are deeply concerned with his welfare. Their goals, if achieved, make the patient better and their own jobs easier. For example, if a bed patient cannot move by himself, the aide or LVN can be taught by the professional how to handle him, benefitting the patient and the staff members. This applies particularly to all of the self-care activities and to movements in the bed.

The entire staff of a nursing home is a team. Each member has a contribution to make, but each one must be able to communicate through the proper chain of command so that everyone knows what the other members are doing. This is where the administrator and the director of nursing have their biggest and most important administrative functions. These administrators are charged with the responsibility of hiring people who are interested in helping the patient of the nursing home. If the employees are truly interested in helping people, then professionals can teach them to achieve the goals of the rehabilitation program.

For these workers to have a chance of success, they must understand the fundamental basis for the patient's rehabilitation:

1. Diagnosis — The physician must give a clear, concise, and definite diagnosis that people unskilled in medicine can understand. If a chart contains the term stroke, this is not a diagnosis; this is a symptom. It may be that the physician cannot make a definite diagnosis. When the patient enters the nursing home, he must get the staff to help him.
2. Plan for prevention of secondary disabilities — A preliminary plan must be started immediately for obvious physical disabilities to prevent secondary problems such as atrophy, contractures, bed sores, etc.
3. A plan for development of functional skills — A person can function in some areas; these areas must be strengthened while working on the impaired areas.
4. Consideration for the dignity of the individual — To help the patients staff members must win their confidence, they must help them gain confidence and develop self-respect. They must be careful how and what they say to patients because they listen to everything.

A rehabilitative program, to be effective, must be fluid, individualized, and guided and supervised by the professionals to see that it is carried out correctly.

GOALS OF REHABILITATION

What does it take to change the outlook of a handicapped person from depression and despair to hopefulness and desire to make a new start in life? It is a technique of rehabilitation that causes the reversal of those biologic tendencies which cause the ill, the disabled, and the elderly to withdraw from life, to deteriorate, and to become dependent. Most elderly handicapped people want to regain their personal independence, and hope to return to their own communities, and wish to find some purpose for living. To achieve these goals, certain ingredients are essential:

1. Patient desire to achieve independence.
2. The proper environment, which has a therapeutic and dynamic approach that encourages recovery.
3. The organization of an overall program of rehabilitation geared to the restoration of function.
4. Wish for personal independence — the abilities to move in bed, to get in and out of bed and from bed to chair, to go to the bathroom, to dress, to wash, and to eat, all without assistance. These are fundamental. There are others who help in personal independence, such as climbing stairs, driving a car, taking care of a home, etc.
5. The need for comprehensive care, which is guidance for return to as useful and satisfying a way of life as possible under the circumstances

Rehabilitation is to restore a person as nearly as possible to the way he was before he was taken ill or disabled. The person who has been affected may have as a goal the restoration to gainful employment. This should then be the goal set by the members of the rehabilitation team. In most cases, the goal of rehabilitation in a nursing home will be to restore the patients to such a state that they are capable of functioning in the society in which they are living. To those who work with the physically disabled, rehabilitation means the complete care of the disabled. Goals and aims in many cases are interchangeable. For example, the aim of rehabilitation for this patient could be the relief of pain and the restoration of function, so by improving mobility and increasing stability, one relieves pain and restores function.

One main problem with understanding rehabilitation is that the whole person is treated for a particular disease by the physician, but the rehabilitation team deals with separate parts of this person. No one treats the whole person. This must be changed.

Many factors need consideration in making goals for patients' rehabilitation. One must consider the duration of the disability, age, ambition, dexterity, gait, intelligence, enthusiasm, and the motivation of the patient. These factors must be added to the reports by all the involved health team members to determine a comprehensive rehabilitative program. Rewards cannot be overlooked as incentives for patients. What will motivate patients to achieve the goals they have set for themselves? The staff team must find what will encourage the patient to want to get well. Thus, the rehabilitation leader must include the education of all the professionals involved in the medical and supportive care to focus endeavors on human values as well as on technical success. The handicapped person needs guidance, understanding, and encouragement to rebuild his life with help from the team. The following functions are important goals in rehabilitation:

1. To gain independence in bed and wheelchair activities
2. To gain maximum use of the extremities
3. To gain the ability to ambulate and elevate
4. To achieve a maximum ability to hear and speak
5. To function in as nearly normal a manner as possible

Keeping these goals in mind, rehabilitation treats the individual in relationship to his family and community. It is an active attitude. It looks for obstacles to overcome for maximum functioning, induces the patient to recognize obstacles, and then tries to motivate the patient to improve these deficiencies. It builds a bridge across the moat that enables him to leave the prison of obstacles. It is a continuing effort to restore function and to reintegrate the patient into his family and community.

The nursing home is the patient's community. The people in it are his family. The nursing home staff can relate the individual to his needs and objectives. Most people need comprehensive care to restore lost or limited functional capacity in order to cope with the environment. This includes prevention of further functional deterioration from the effects of an existing disability. Thus, medical rehabilitation is the clinical process by which the disabled person is restored to a state of optimal effectiveness and is given an opportunity to enjoy a meaningful life.

Rehabilitation, by definition, is committed to restoring, improving, or maintaining functional abilities — emotional and social adjustment that patients may develop to their fullest extent. For a rehabilitative program to have meaning it must be realistic. It must be geared to the patient's personality, to his physical and mental capacity, and must satisfy his desire for living. If rehabilitation ignores these realities, it will never achieve its goals, which should also be the patient's. Some personalities of patients, such as the overdependent and the resigned patient, hinder or make it impossible to obtain the desired goals.

These considerations are especially essential when working with the elderly patient. The medical team that does not have the primary and secondary goals accompanied by appropriate measures will not be successful with the elderly patient. The aid of all health professional available must be enlisted, which will result in increased functional activity for the patient. Older people can profit by using staff personnel to improve their restorative goals and to live a more fruitful and healthier life.

One of the major problems is the medical and nursing traditional negative attitudes towards the elderly patient. Such attitudes are unrealistic in light of the demonstrated capacity of elderly patients to profit by restorative rehabilitation resulting in a more meaningful life. The professional attitude towards the aged, disabled, and chronically ill patient has been characterized, in general, by a premature resignation to the inevitability of decline and a patronizing attitude that basically reflects the uneasiness of the physician who recognizes his own helplessness in the situation and is reminded of his own mortality. The needs of the aged disabled people go beyond the bare necessities of food, shelter, and medical care.

REHABILITATION AND THE AGED

A large percentage of our elderly, disabled patients have gradually accumulated many minor disabling conditions, as a result of a primary disability. In many cases, these secondary conditions need to be treated before, or at the same time as, the primary one in order to achieve any degree of rehabilitation. The members of a rehabilitation team can only function if the patient can participate fully in the program. Careful attention to the minor medical details of these patients may well provide the key to the successful rehabilitation.

Keep in mind the definition of rehabilitation. As stated before, it is safe to say that the aged person with an impairment is a handicapped one who has a disability. Restorative goals must be realistic. A key thought that must be kept in mind is the energies of both patient and staff should be directed towards those areas offering greatest potential for independence and improvement. The staff's basic aim should be the correction of that condition which provokes the greatest frustration to the patient.

REHABILITATIVE PROGRAM

Long-Term Rehabilitation

When talking about long-range goals for the elderly, disabled, and handicapped patient, one should include the following:

1. Reasonable functional improvements
2. Maintenance of existing abilities
3. Retardation of deterioration
4. Prevention of secondary complications

Daily Short-Term Rehabilitation

The staff must be reminded that the patient must want to be helped; otherwise, they can do very little for him. Factors tending to limit cooperation may be physical or emotional. Thus, mobility and personal independence can be hampered by frustration, distortion of self-image, and the insecurity the new environment creates.

The following approach on a day-to-day basis is effective:

1. Create a stimulating atmosphere
2. Provide an opportunity for the patient to overcome obstacles. This will result in cooperation which would lead to the patient trying to solve his own problems.

The itemized activities of the program must be professional and individualized. They must be firm, flexible, and understanding.

REHABILITATION STATUS

Attention to the rehabilitative aspects of care from the earliest possible moment implies a continuity of service and avoidance of any break between acute, convalescent, and rehabilitation management. It should be emphasized that delay in institution of rehabilitation is costly in terms of time and money.

Rehabilitation is a medical discipline. The initial development of modern rehabilitation and its rapid evolution occurred principally in large rehabilitation centers, many supported by grants and public funds. The organizations and the interrelationships of rehabilitation teams vary from place to place, and as a result there is poor coordination in some cases. In the course of an evaluation, several physicians may first study the patient, then the physical therapist, the occupational therapist, the speech therapist, the psychologist, social worker, and, finally, a recreational therapist make evaluations. They all meet, and if each feels his evaluation is the most important, it results in the patient's being subjected to complicated and fractionated treatment, which causes a costly delay in rehabilitation.

In the interest of the patient and efficiency, it is essential that priorities be given to certain phases of rehabilitation and that others be postponed until the patient is ready. For each phase, this simplest approach should be used. Nonessential diagnostic procedures should be postponed. Emphasis should be placed on the development of standardized technical procedures that will lead to the desired goals. The use of group methods of exercise is desirable because it spares personnel and also adds the element of competition that raises morale.

One of the major obstacles to rehabilitation has been the lack of funds to support the treatment of the disabled. The money available for rehabilitation has been distributed very unevenly. Only in recent years has there been any money available for rehabilitation of the elderly, disabled, and dependent patients. A great many handicapped people exhaust their financial resources and have nowhere to turn for support.

There are three phases to medical care: (1) prevention, (2) medical or surgical care, and (3) rehabilitation.

If rehabilitation is understood to encompass prevention of disabilities as well as maintenance of maximal physical function and emotional balance during the course of definitive treatment, it is obvious that rehabilitation must begin in parallel with the definitive medical care rather than at the end of the prevention, medical, or surgical phase.

The patient who requires rehabilitation services must maintain a relationship with medical services whether provided by the hospital or in the nursing home. Whenever possible, rehabilitation should be carried out as a continuing program with general medical care. Regardless of the location of the services, there should be a good liaison and communications between those directing the rehabilitation and the physician.

The person in need of rehabilitation needs both medical and psychosocial services. The two aspects of rehabilitation, namely, physical re-education or strengthening and psychosocial adjustment, must go hand in hand. The physician, with the help of a physical therapist in addition to a good social worker with access to community resources, forms a working partnership for the patient's benefit. This is the framework for a very satisfactory rehabilitation team.

If one assumes that a major disability is handled best in a well-staffed nursing home or convalescent center or extended care facility, the course of events should be somewhat as follows:

1. Diagnostic evaluation study that analyzes the problem and provides a basis for program planning and a preliminary prognosis.
2. A therapeutic program scheduled according to priorities of goals and consistent with the patient's interests and capabilities.
3. Concurrent psychosocial service aimed at utilizing family or community relationships, securing economic resources, and exploiting interests, attitudes, and aptitudes that can lead the disabled person back into the normal stream of activity.
4. Planning for discharge, a joint enterprise of the medical and psychosocial staff, preferably initiated early and developed in close cooperation with the patient.
5. Follow up observation.

PRINCIPLES OF REHABILITATION

Rehabilitation in its widest sense signifies the whole process of restoring a disabled person to a condition in which he is able, as early as possible, to resume a normal life.

Rehabilitation is creative convalescence, and, as such, represents the active contribution made by medical professionals, allied health staff, and the patient to the restoration of health during the recovery period followed by the intensive definite treatment.

Planned rehabilitation must start soon after the onset of the disability. The advantage of organized rehabilitation lies in its ability to combine the medical and functional assessment into an integrated program for the benefit of the patient, thus enabling the patient's rehabilitation to progress smoothly without unnecessary delays.

The foundation of good rehabilitation lies in good medicine. This is manifested by accurate diagnosis, careful prognosis, and early, appropriate, and adequate definite care. The superstructure of rehabilitation depends considerably upon the bricks of physical therapy, the rehabilitative nurse, the nursing service, the recreational therapist, and social service.

Unfortunately, responsibilities tend to become separated, and it becomes necessary to have one person bring about the integration of the entire team. This integration calls for good organization and management and clearly defined lines of communication and areas of responsibility. Nursing homes that provide rehabilitation must find such a person to head up this area to make it successful. The person's title is not important; the end result is what counts.

The person in charge of rehabilitation must give his staff the following instructions to achieve the results that he desires:

1. An accurate diagnosis
2. Clear indications of the aims of treatment for each patient
3. A clear indication of the likely outcome
4. Specifications where drug therapy or disease characteristics may necessitate particular care in the administration of various treatments.

This person should remember that short, intensive periods of therapy are more likely to have a therapeutic value than the prolonged, intermittent attendances for palliative treatment, which rapidly becomes more of a social outing than a therapeutic activity. He should encourage the team members to record details of the nature and effect of treatment so that feedback information from their trained observations may substantially influence future management and enable them to contribute fully to its outcome.

TECHNIQUES OF REHABILITATION

1. Physical measures such as active and passive exercises, positioning

2. Mechanical devices such as braces, splints, prosthesis, wheelchairs, crutches, canes, and self-help devices
3. Education, counseling, social service, psychological help

To carry out the rehabilitation technique, the staff needs —

1. a diagnosis that determines the pathological status;
2. an evaluation of functional status and estimate of potential improvement:
   a. Test for muscular strength and contractures
   b. Measure of joint mobility
   c. Test for endurance
3. a statement of desired improvements in physical, mental, and social functions.

The usual complaints of patients are as follows:

1. Lack of mobility, in part or as a whole
2. Pain in certain areas, at rest or upon movement
3. Feeling of neglect

Routines for restitution of physical function:

1. For those patients confined to bed routines are as follows:
   a. Suitability of the mattress and the bed
   b. Positioning
      (1) Type of mattress
      (2) Safety precautions
      (3) Use of sandbags and footboard
   c. Type of exercise for the bed patient
      (1) Range of motion (ROM)
      (2) Stretching contractures
      (3) Muscle setting (isometric exercise)
2. Use of tilt table, transfer activities, ambulation, and activities of daily living. The latter includes elevation activities, such as sitting, and need for a support, such as sling, brace, cane, or crutches.
3. Range of motion: All joints possess their own ranges; this is the area though which they are able to move, such as bending the knee joint. Moving various joints though their ranges of motion once or twice a day may prevent tightening or stiffening and functional loss. Again, it is important not to force or try to speed up this activity. Extra care is required when moving a joint below

a tighter joint, as in trying to move a tight shoulder by rotating the forearm. This could strain the elbow and perhaps nearby structures. The movement through a simple range of motion is an art.

4. Rest: Failure to include purposeful rest can result in failure of any exercise or function program. Staff must make it clear that it is important to rest between exercises. Before, after, and between individual exercises. Rest and relaxation must be practiced. At the beginning of the functional program of self-care, it is important to make the program relatively short. Muscles must rest, and muscles must work to function properly.

5. Frequency of exercising: To start with, the exercises for groups or individuals should be done once a day. Development for more exercise periods will depend on many factors and relate to the individual participating.

The program is geared to the patient's improvement and motivation. Nearly every patient wants to improve. Build on that for motivation. The worker must have the proper philosophy in order to achieve good results.

GENERAL PRINCIPLES OF RESTORATIVE CARE

Once principles of rehabilitation have been established, the creativity of the trained individuals on the rehabilitation team can be applied:

1. Definite diagnosis
2. Prevention of secondary disability
3. Development of functional abilities
4. Preservation of the dignity of the individual

Staff members must be able to instill in the patient self-respect and confidence in his abilities.

Concepts of Restorative Care

Due to improved communication between the health professionals and the general public, there is a new awareness in the development of restorative techniques, which makes people realize that physical disability need no longer be looked upon as a hopeless

condition. It must be remembered that crippling disease not only affect a patient's physical health but also have far-reaching emotional,
social, and economic complications, all of which result in difficulties
in integrating these people into the community. Rehabilitation aims
to correct these deficiencies to a degree that would ultimately assure
maximal independence within the limits of the patient's disability.
Rehabilitation is a complex activity, and it has been defined as a
philosophy, an objective, and a method. The philosophy is the
strong conviction that every patient, even the most severely disabled, has considerable physical and emotional resources. Furthermore, a conscious refusal to accept defeat in the belief that these patients, if properly managed and mobilized, can again resume a com-
paratively well-adjusted existence in the community outside the institution will achieve results.

Since the primary object of rehabilitation is to create optimal
health and social conditions, there is a need for comprehensive
rehabilitation. Comprehensive rehabilitation is a multidisciplinary
activity to which a variety of professionals contribute the knowledge
and skills of their own specialties. This field is termed restorative
because each specialty, from physician to every member of the team,
contributes to the restoration of the patient. At present, conventional medicine encourages disease-centered specialization, whereas
a restorative program goes far beyond the elimination of the disease
and endeavors to solve patients' problems on a more comprehensive
level. It recognizes the importance of emotional, social, economic,
and other environmental factors concomitant with physical restoration.

REHABILITATIVE NURSING

The role of a nurse is a complex one because in a rehabilitative
setting nurses must in part render a higher type of comprehensive
patient care. They must work with many disciplines that make up
the rehabilitation team. In rehabilitation nursing, nurses are practi-
tioners, educators, coordinators, and leaders of the rehabilitation
team all at once. Much depends on their relationships to other allied
health groups and their abilities to identify all aspects of a patient's
disabilities and keep them in proper perspective. The nursing service
renders an essential and unique contribution to the overall health

services needed to restore the patient to his maximal functional capacity. This is only achieved by twenty-four-hour nursing care of the patient.

Nursing standards must be set, nursing care of the patient maintained, and the nursing program planned and carried out. Rehabilitation nurses are usually, or should be, heads of the rehabilitation team. On the whole, they will analyze the nursing service required to evaluate the quality of nursing service provided by all nursing personnel and study methods to improve patient care by encouraging the practice of rehabilitative principles in every nursing situation. They are the educators, being responsible for the orientation of new staff, and active in-service training program directors. They are administrators to hire qualified, competent, and motivated people capable of carrying out the principles of patient care in relationship to the rehabilitation needs of the patients. Under the direction of the nursing service are the staff nurses, practical nurses, licensed vocational nurses, nurses' aides, and volunteers; these people are the heart of patient care. These are the people who work twenty-four hours a day with the patients. They must be motivated and dedicated. They can make a success or failure of the goals.

Each team member needs to work closely with every other. To obtain greater insight and understanding regarding patient's needs, each team member must relate to all others on the team in such a way that opinions and ideas are easily exchanged, information is traded, and help and advice are given when needed. It must be a two-way street. It is important to remember that the fundamental idea in all rehabilitation is that a person is a total being — that he is composed of physical, mental, and social entities that constitute a whole.

PATIENT CARE

Patient care is a written plan of nursing care. Planning is the answer to quality nursing programs. The first thing the staff must do is to decide on the form that they will use. Different patients will have different information because of their needs. It is essential that one person be responsible for filling out the details of the form, especially if the patient is assisting. Remember that patients' needs

are unmet for a varitey of reasons but primarily due to lack of information. Incorrect needs are identified due to the lack of patient participation. The nurse needs to seek facts and relate them to the patient's needs. What method does the nurse use to get information
essential to making a plan to help the patient? Does she involve the
patient? Does she talk to the patient's family? Is it through direct
questions, observations, informal conversations, and planned conferences? What do other members of the rehabilitation team contribute?

Physiological, psychological, and social areas are the three main
assessments of the patient. The initial start should include the
following:

1. Medical diagnosis
2. General condition of the patient
3. Detailed observations of the particular condition
4. Observations of the nurse, LVN, aide, and specialists on the
   rehabilitation team
5. Patient's attitude
6. Family attitude

Many institutions have as a start a chart called *Admission Interview*
sometimes called *Nursing History*. Following is a sample:

Admission Interview

Patient's Name:
Date:
Height: Weight: Age:

Questions:

Have you ever been in a nursing home before? If yeş, tell me about
it.

What are you here for? Goals or objectives.

Do you have any problems sleeping? If yes, do you have any
medication for it?

Are you on a special diet? If yes, what is it? Any special medication?

Do you have any eating problems? Using tools, dentures, others?

Do you have any hearing or visual problems? Glasses or hearing aids?

Do you have any problems with your bowels? Do you have any medication?

What family do you have? Who is close by?

Do you expect visitors? Phone calls? Do you want to go out?

Do you have any questions about the nursing home?

Did you choose to come to this home?

Did you visit the nursing home before you came to stay?

Tell me anything that will help me to give you the best of care while you are here.

While interviewing the patient, the nurse should note such facts as what the patient's attitude is, how anxious the patient is, whether he is fearful of coming to the facility, whether he discussed this family, what type of speech he has and what his facial expression is. There should be space for the interviewer's impressions and any notes he wants to make, for example, questions that the patient did not or could not answer.

Nurses have a difficult situation when they are confronted with a new admission to the nursing home. The patient may come in at a time that is not appropriate, e.g. when they are very busy with a sick patient. A new admission may come with a large number of family members. The patient may come in unexpectedly, perhaps the staff was not informed. The patient may come in when the nurse has a personnel problem that needs to be resolved. What should be done? In addition, there are people who have certain illnesses or handicaps that influence nurses in certain ways. Also, people may make snap judgments upon meeting a new patient. Most important, the staff must watch themselves due to prejudices. This is something that is conditioned by environment, socioeconomic life, and family traditions. Experience develops nurses into realizing some of their reactions, and as they improve and become better people, their associates and patients will notice. They will find that they can do a better job with their patients, which is the primary concern.

Nursing Care Plan is Part of Patient Care

There are five basic steps in drawing up plans for patients:

1. Collection of data
2. Identification of problems
3. Tentative approach to the problem
4. Evaluation on how effective the plan is
5. Changing or adjusting the plan due to continuous evaluations

It is important that all members who are working on a particular patient make notes on the patient's chart after they finish working with him. Thus, all will share in the observations and conclusions of the members of the team.

Suggested Nursing Care Plan

Admission date   Tolerance
Diagnosis   Allergies
                                                     Diet
Independence code: Bath facilities
  I — Independence
  S — Supervise
  D — Dependent
  A — Assist

Activities of daily living	Medications		Appliances
Bed activities	Date	Stop Date	Wheelchair (how often)
Bed positioning — supine			Braces
prone			Others
side			
Transfers	Treatments:		Discharge planning
Upper dressing	R.O.M.		Family instructions
Lower dressing	Positioning		Diet
Feet	Transfer		Welfare referral
Bladder program	activities		Health agency
Bowel program	Others		Futher instructions
suppository			Equipment needed
stimulation			
Daily hygiene			
Bed			
Bathing			
Feeding			
Family			
Special interests			
General attitude			

Temporary goals
Long-range goals

Special area of emphasis

Age: Room: Physician in Charge:

The Nurse and Nursing Service

The physician's examination of the patient, followed by orders for medication and treatment is the first step. The nurse and nursing service then takes over and must check the following:

1. Must see to such hygienic factors as bath, oral hygiene, shaving, care of hair, cleanliness, condition of the nails (hands and feet).
2. The environment is part of the staff's responsibility, such things as heat control, noise, roommates, care of patient's personal items.
3. What assistance does the patient need? Meals, ambulation, dressing, communication.
4. Safety factors.
5. The nurse must plan to see that —
   a. the patient is in proper alignment in bed;
   b. no circulatory problems are present;
   c. infection is prevented;
   d. contractures are prevented;
   e. there is relief from pain;
   f. elements for elimination are accessible;
   g. psychological support is available;
   h. church attendance is possible, if desired;
   i. other members of the team study, test, and evaluate the new patient.

The nursing service and members of the rehabilitation team working with a patient must be careful of their evaluation. All members of the team must have their evaluations using the same factors in their judgments. It is important in the evaluation to consider the following:

1. Bed Activities: Can the patient move from side to side; can they come to a sitting position by themselves?
2. Positioning: Does the patient need to be in the supine, prone,

or side-lying position? How long and what hours? Turning schedule? What skin problems exist?

3. Range of Motion (R.O.M.): What extremities require R.O.M.? What special precautions are required?

4. Transfers: Can the patient get in and out of bed? To the wheelchair, toilet, tub, automobile? Does he stand or sit to transfer?

5. Dressing:
    a. Can patients dress the upper part of their bodies?
    b. Can they dress the lower part of their bodies?
    c. Can they manage after the toilet?
    d. What kind of shoes and stockings do they use?
    e. Are they using braces?
    f. Can they put on their own braces?
    g. Do they have any bandages?

6. Bladder Program:
    a. Does the patient have a Foley catheter, a leg bag?
    b. What is the schedule for irrigation of the catheter or general voiding?

7. Bowel Program:
    a. What schedule is planned?
    b. Are medications and suppositories used?

8. Daily Hygiene:
    a. Can they bathe themselves?
    b. Can they brush their teeth?
    c. Can they care for their dentures?
    d. What about general grooming?

9. Locomotion:
    a. Wheelchair — hand propelled or motorized?
    b. Ambulation — independent, walker, crutches, cane or canes?
    c. Gait?
    d. Can they use stairs or steps?

10. Feeding:
    a. Do they need help?
    b. Do they use dentures?
    c. Do they use any adaptive equipment?
    d. Are they on a special diet?

11. Vision:
    a. Do they have impaired vision?
    b. Do they wear glasses?
12. Hearing:
    a. Are the patients hearing impaired?
    b. Do they wear aids?
    c. Do they lip-read?
    d. Can they hear better from one side than the other?
13. Speech:
    a. Can they write?
    b. Do they understand words?
    c. Do they understand when spoken to?
    d. Do they understand writing?
    e. Have they any speech problems?
    f. Do they only speak a foreign lanuage?
14. Mental Ability:
    a. Are they alert?
    b. Are they forgetful?
    c. Do they have periods of confusion?
    d. Are they comatose?
    e. What kind of learning do they have?
    f. Do they learn quickly?
       (1) Do they require repetitive teaching?
       (2) Is demonstration necessary?
       (3) Are they unable to learn?
15. Psychological Approach:
    a. Does the patient need encouragement?
    b. Do they need restricting?
    c. Do they follow through with learned activities?
    d. What are some of their goals that might give clues in helping them?
16. Discharge Plan:
    a. Is there one?
    b. Is there a need for one?
    c. What family instructions have been given?
    d. Has the patient gone home overnight?
    e. Has a public health referral been made?
    f. Has the welfare agency been notified, if necessary?

g. What equipment will be needed and has it been ordered?

The patient does not necessarily have to be someone who is very ill or handicapped. However, the person with a medical problem is often the one whose need for regimen of activity and/or exercise is overlooked. The more serious the illness, it seems, the greater the likelihood that such a program will be unduly delayed. The patient that has had a medical or surgical disability is often advised to be up, but spends most of that time in a chair with little real activity. It usually contributes to poor comfort or poor posture. Exercise is often an attitude as well as an activity and has much to offer the patient for rehabilitation. A proper exercise program merges the physical and behavioral care. Denial is often seen in patients, particularly in those who have suffered a stroke and have lost movement and some vision on one side. As patients becomes aware become aware of improvement, they; gain psychological support, feeling that they are just taking pills. The patient must be constantly reminded of the greater rewards that proper activity can bring.

In many cases, the nursing home patient is often the most difficult to deal with because of immobilization. This situation should be changed as quickly as the patient's medical or surgical problem will permit and should not be overlooked by the nursing staff or rehabilitation team. More attention is being given to patients who are immobilized because of the likelihood of irreparable damage. It is now recognized that lack of exercise is an important risk in heart disease. Patients who have suffered cerebral vascular accidents or who have undergone complex joint replacements are now frequently out of bed within hours. Experience in cardiology has shown that it is advisable to have a person with uncomplicated myocardial infarction taking active therapeutic exercises within a few days, thereby reducing anxiety and psychophysiologic stress. Failure to use muscles is tantamount to abusing muscles because they are made to function and will atrophy if not used. Any illness that requires immobilzation or confinement to bed for long periods of time will most certainly devitalize the patient. A disturbance of the functions in even one joint may upset a large part of the entire muscular system.

The effect of bed may be compared to that of a drug, useful in the correct amount but harmful in overdosage or in excess. It is safe to say that improving function on one side of the body may lead to improved function on the other side. This also applies to related joints and muscles.

Patient Education and Motivation

Patients are now an enlightened and interested group, but they are likely to have an incomplete and unbalanced accumulation of medical knowledge. This means that the rehabilitation team must inform patients more fully concerning the aspects of their particular needs. This is especially true in the therapeutic exercises because patients are expected to assume some responsiblility for their own improvement. There is a growing awareness within medicine and rehabilitation for more health care education for the patient and the family. This enhances the delivery of better health care and certainly lessens the expense. There must be a partnership between the members of the rehabilitation team, the physician, and the nursing home staff with the patient. This would lead to better health management. As patients learn to practice all of their rehabilitative activities, they soon realize that functional activity development is vital to their health and well-being. Meaningful activities that can be understood and accomplished must be patterned for them.

Motivation is a very important factor in health care. It goes in concert with understanding, education, and faith in self and the people working with them. It also means that the patient has hope. Most patients want to improve physically but may lack incentive. Motivation can be aroused and supported by the proper rehabilitation program and by having the right people work with them.

One of the latest methods used for motiviation is the group therapy method. It is a new experience both for the leader and for the patient. The group may be of any size, but the therapy can and must be personalized with individual attention to each participant. Groups may be formed of patients with pulmonary problems, cardiovascular troubles, diabetes, and other medical conditions. In the treatments of stroke, patients are grouped while the patients are in certain stages of disability and progress. Each specialist can come to this group and work with them, as this reduces the cost of specialized care. It is very difficult to measure the amount of stimulation that this type of activity contributes to the patient's development. However, it has been proven that group therapy is one of the best means of arousing patient motivation. Patients for the first time find that they are not alone with their particular type of disability, and this helps them to develop a constructive attitude. Progress is regularly seen and measured when patients join together in a common goal of personal improvement. Most patients who see others as ill as they are, and with similar problems, become less likely to indulge in self-pity. They acquire a more realistic view of their problems and derive satisfaction and reassurance from being with others with whom they have much in common. Often one person will try to do better than another, particularly in an exercise program and the competition becomes very keen. A benefit of group therapy is the companionship that it provides. In many instances, members of the family are allowed to participate. The purpose of this is for the interested members of the family to learn what happens in therapy and to get involved with their family member in doing activities together. This gives them a better understanding of the problems that confront the patient in regaining his physical and mental strength.

FUNDAMENTALS AND PRECAUTIONS CONCERNING ACTIVITIES

It is of utmost importance that each member of the rehabilitation team be aware of patients' needs as expressed in their medical records. Staff members must see that patients understand the program, that the activities are taught properly, and that patients learn and understand each step of the exercise or functional self-care activity. The basic principles can be easily learned and should be adapted to fit each individual's health problem. Rapid improvement with improved independence often depends on the correctness and energy of training during each session:

WARM–UP. It is essential for patients to be prepared for their exercise program.

PROPER CLOTHING. In some cases, proper clothing is of no consequence; in others it is of the utmost importance. Clothing must be comfortable. If the patient is to get out of bed, the proper shoes must be available. Clothing must not hinder the process of getting in or out of bed.

MENTAL ATTITUDE. The patient should be encouraged to think of the benefits of the program and have faith in what it can do. Mental readiness is necessary. A good attitude is needed for achievement. Yet, at the same time, the patient must understand that they are to do what they can, what is reasonable, without getting fatigued.

RESTRICTIONS. Movements should not be forced. If there are restrictions in any joint or muscle, do not strain this activity.

SPEED OF MOVEMENT. There is usually an optimal speed of motion for each muscle and joint group. Moving too slowly may be a waste of time, but moving too fast can cause a muscle strain and imbalance. A natural speed should be sought. Start the movements slowly and smoothly and stop easily.

THE PHYSICIAN AND REHABILITATION

The practice of rehabilitation for any physician begins with belief in the basic philosophy that the physician's responsibility does not end when the acute illness is ended or surgery is completed; it ends only when the patient is retrained to live and work with what is left. This basic concept of the physician's responsibility can be achieved only if rehabilitation is considered an integral part of medical service. Any program of rehabilitation is only as sound as the basic medical service of which it is a part. The diagnosis and prognosis must be accurate, for it is upon them that the feasibility of retraining is determined. In addition to the general diagnostic studies, the medical evaluation of the handicapped patient must include (1) muscle tests, (2) range of motion, and (3) tests for daily living activities.

In making a checklist to get the information to help in an evaluation, the staff should check the following:

1. Bed activities
   a. Moving from place to place in bed
   b. Ability to sit erect
2. Toilet activities
3. Eating and drinking
4. Ability to dress and undress
   a. Tying shoelaces
   b. Pulling up zippers

    c. Buttoning shirt
    d. Putting on and taking off a brace
5. Hand activities
    a. Winding a watch
    b. Striking a match
    c. Using and turning a doorknob
6. Wheelchair activities
    a. Getting from the bed to the wheelchair, from wheelchair to bed
7. Elevation Activities
    a. Needed abilities for walking, climbing, and traveling

The physician need not do these tests himself. A well-trained rehabilitative nurse or a physical therapist can do it for him. There are fundamental procedures that he must know. He must recommend certain rehabilitative steps. To illustrate these procedures or steps, let us take a patient who is hemiplegic as a result of a stroke. In the early stages of treatment and rehabilitation, the following procedures should be instituted to prevent deformities caused by contractures:

    1. Footboard or posterior leg splint to prevent foot drop.
    2. Sandbags to prevent outward rotation of the affected leg.
    3. A pillow in the axilla to prevent adduction of the shoulder.
    4. Quadriceps setting to maintain strength.

The next procedure is the use of a pulley if a trapeze bar is not available. This is done by attaching a small pulley to a goose-neck pipe over the door of the room, using a clothesline with a webbing at the end for a hand loop. With the stretching and pulling provided by this pulley, the range of motion can be increased, and adhesions and atrophy prevented. The advantage of the pulley over passive stretching exercises is that the patient does the stretching and will only go as far as the pain threshold allows. The pulley also can be used in motion patterns. At this stage, the patient should be encouraged to sit erect in order to re-establish balance.

Speech therapy, if needed, should be started at this point.

If the facility does not have a trained speech therapist, then a teacher who is interested, under the training of the physician, can give the training to the patient. It is well for the physician to point out to the family and the patient the nature of his condition. Loss of

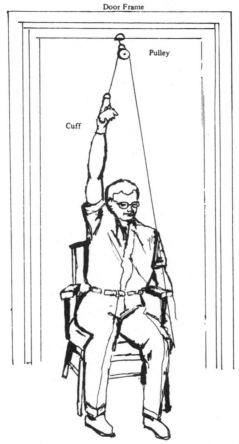

Figure 6-1. Patient in chair in front of door using pulley with webbing to do range of motion exercises.

the ability to use the tools of communication must not be interpreted as a loss or diminution of the ability to think and reason.

The next step in the rehabilitation of the stroke patient is ambulation:

1. The patient should practice balance in the standing position, then move to the parallel bars; if bars are not available, then he should use two kitchen chairs to balance himself.
2. A short leg brace will be needed in approximately ½ of all cases, with an ankle stop to help prevent a foot drop.
3. A heel and toe gait should be taught to minimize clonus and to

re-establish normal walking habits, stressing reciprocal motion.

4. Instruction in crutch walking, then begins, usually the four-point gait.

5. Finally there is a teaching elevation, stressing climbing steps, curbs, etc.

Throughout rehabilitation as concurrent training, the nursing service must carry out the functions of self-care and daily living activities. It is obvious that the physician cannot undertake the rehabilitation program; it is his responsibility to see that the program is carried out by a qualified physical therapist. It is his duty to provide all the necessary care for the best interests of his patient. This is just one example of how the physician and rehabilitation staff can work together for the best interests of the physician's patients.

In rehabilitation, the primary consideration in working out a program for severely handicapped individuals is to teach them to improve what is left, and to accept their limitations with equanimity. Too frequently, in rehabilitation, many of the basic skills necessary for effective daily living are overlooked. The patient is given numerous medical, psychological, and social tests, but rehabilitation in the basic physical skills of ambulation, elevation, and self-care activities of daily living is neglected, resulting in the inability of patients to walk, travel, or care for their personal needs and the inability to utilize effectively the medical, psychological, and social services they have received.

Rehabilitation in the basic physical skills of daily living is primary. It is simply a matter of "first things first." Daily activity skills are the basis for all subsequent rehabilitation processes. It has been found difficult, in many instances, to differentiate between muscular inability due to disease and that due to atrophy of disuse. Tests must be made, and then a suitable program must be set up for individuals to meet their particular needs.

The physician must recognize that emotional trauma may be present in any patient who has suffered a severe physical disability. The sudden shock and realization of the possible economic and social sequences of permanent disability frequently produce fear and anxiety, which become as handicapping to the individual as the original physical disability. It is the responsibility of the physician to recognize the need for psychological help and to see that proper referrals are made for this problem. In some instances where emotional problems are of a less severe nature the physician can resolve these problems himself. One of the greatest problems the physician has with patients that have severe physical handicaps is motivation. He must encourage and convince patients that they can be rehabilitated.

For this motivation to be most effective, it must begin at the earliest possible moment following the accident or illness. The physician who knows something about rehabilitation can start at the time of the accident or disease to allay the fears of his patient. This is accomplished by giving him understanding, courage, and hope predicated on an accurate knowledge of what can be done. He can interpret to the patient the findings of the specialists in words that are understandable and meaningful. He can explain to the patient the nature and extent of his disability, not only in medical terms of the disability, but the effects it will have on his family, his economics, and his social life. The physician must practice the art of medicine as well as the science.

Regardless of the type of disability, the responsibility of the physician to his patients cannot end when the acute injury has been treated. It ends only when the physician has made certain that proper referrals have been made to those agencies and institutions which are equipped to rehabilitate patients to their fullest restoration.

The physician who fails to see that those patients under their care receive the full benefits of modern methods of rehabilitation is in the same category as the physician who still persists in using dietary restrictions alone in the management of diabetes when insulin is available. Medical care is not complete until patients have been trained to live and work with their remaining ability.

MAINTENANCE CARE

There are many patients so damaged beyond medical assistance that full rehabilitation is out of the question. Perhaps the only therapeutic efforts would be at least to delay deterioration and prevent unnecessary disability and suffering. Thus, the nursing home's purpose is clear in having a maintenance program. It may be very little more than periodic turning in bed to prevent disuse, or it may require special methods of feeding. Whatever the nature of the irremediable defects and regardless of the degree of disability, there is always something to be done to make life more tolerable, if not for the patients, at least for their families and friends, who also suffer.

Rehabilitation practices with elderly patients have demonstrated the enormous needs that prevail. Patients that fall into the class of geriatric rehabilitation have been classified by Dasco (1953) into three principal groups:

1. The obviously handicapped person, such as hemiplegia, arthritis, fractures, amputations.
2. The chronically ill patient without signs of a manifest disability, such as a chronic organic condition, cardiac disease, pulmonary disease, etc.
3. The elderly person who is not obviously ill but whose physical fitness is impaired.

There is no reason why all of the three classes do not receive rehabilitation. The importance of early rehabilitation can hardly be overemphasized, since the conditions of patients in each of the groups tend to deteriorate rapidly in the absence of proper care. Restoration of maximum function is the goal for people of all ages. The elderly person's maximum functioning may mean an adjustment to the demands of daily living activities and psychologic adjustment. In most elderly patients, however, self-sufficiency in ambulating, washing, eating, dressing, and toileting activities is the primary goal. If patients have attained the maximum performance in these areas, as well as made the best psychosocial adjustment possible for themselves, then rehabilitative goals have been successful. The challenge is self-sufficiency.

Thus, goals for rehabilitation of elderly patients must be constantly adjusted to their needs as ascertained for them in their environment. This applies to the time allowed for specific gains, as well as to the final objectives. Retraining for activities for daily living is a primary goal due to the patient's condition. Living can be successfully provided if there is appropriate modification in both tempo and goals. This is particularly important, since transfer from a wheelchair to the bed or toilet, eating, dressing, and washing are significant contributions to the older person's comfort and efficiency as well as to those who would otherwise have to carry out or assist them with such functions.

The prevention of disability is always preferable to its alleviation or cure. Patterns of living that originate in middle age and go until end of life such as proper diet, safety precaution, freedom from excessive physical and emotional strains, adequate income, satisfying social and recreational activities are all essential for ensuring health in later years. The extremely important steps are the early detection and, if possible, elimination of any form of disease or adjustment. The teaching of health habits and health information as it affects older people should be clear and practical. Proper nutrition and dental care should be maintained in the elderly person. Malnutrition is frequently related to denial, blaming dentures, for example.

What elderly people need is a mode of life that will allow them to prevent, or at least postpone, the occurrence of disabling chronic disease.

In chronic illness, efforts at prevention are not as successful as in an infectious disease. The main tool in forestalling severe complications of chronic disease is their early discovery. This fact has been realized by authorities in the field of preventive medicine and public health. The sources of many disabling chronic diseases can be traced back to simple origins, at which point appropriate countermeasures could have prevented their full development.

In the dietary regime, there is no specific menu designed for the elderly person. The diet prescribed for an elderly person should be geared to individual physiologic and pathologic requirements. It is not age but the disease that should determine the patient's prescription for dietary needs. It is interesting to note that in reviewing elderly patient's eating habits it reveals that fads prevail rather than the need for proper nutrition; thus, the essential food elements are curtailed. To follow dietary fads, or to use nutritional additives unnecessarily as older persons sometimes do, might lead to an unbalanced and insufficient diet.

Physical activity is strongly indicated for the elderly patient. The beneficial effects that are derived from proper and appropriate activities are real to the participants. Each person must take an active interest and participate in his own life and those around him as well.

It is particularly important that people who work in nursing homes should be temperamentally suited to and interested in working with older people. Rehabilitation workers should always be carefully chosen because the work with the elderly disabled patients places a special demand on the patience and maturity of people dealing with them. It has been proven that in the absence of suitable personnel, the care and treatment of the elderly patient degenerates into apathy and neglect.

In rehabilitation, one is dealing with physical, psychological, social, economic, and vocational components of a person's life. In order for rehabilitation to be effective, it must begin as early as possible. Rehabilitation is a creative process that allows maximal use of existing abilities. The patient and his family are essential members of the team of health workers that will make it possible for rehabilitation to have a permanent effect on the patient's life after the actual medical program has ended. In conclusion, a realistic definition of rehabilitation was made by Doctor Paul M. Ellwood in a speech, in which he says, "Rehabilitation is basically an optimistic process which concedes that despite continuing and even catastrophic disability, a better way of life for the patient is possible."

REFERENCES

1. *Rehabilitation and Medicine,* by Sidney Licht. Waverly Press, Baltimore, Maryland, 1968.
2. *Handbook of Physical Medicine and Rehabilitation,* by the Council on Physical Medicine and Rehabilitation, A.M.A. The Blakiston Co., Philadelphia, Pennsylvania, 1950.
3. Essays on Rehabilitation, by Howard Rusk. In *Handbook of Physical Medicine and Rehabilitation,* A.M.A. The Blakiston Co., Philadelphia, Pennsylvania, 1950.
4. *Rehabilitation,* by Gerald G. Hirshberg, Leon Lewis, and Dorothy Thomas. J.B. Lippencott Co., Philadelphia, Pennsylvania, 1964.
5. *Rehabilitation Medicine,* by P.J.R. Nichols. Butterworths, London, 1976.
6. Clinical Problems in Geriatric Rehabilitation, by M.M. Dasco. *Geriatrics,* 8:179, April, 1953.
7. *Aging,* by N.W. Shock. Some Social and Biological Aspects, Pub. No. 65, Washington, D.C. 1960.
8. *Rehabilitation Nursing,* by A.B. Morrissey, G.P. Putnam's Sons, New York, 1951.
9. *Nursing in Rehabilitation,* National League for Nursing, Bibliography, New York, 1955.
10. *Rehabilitation Aspects of Acute and Chronic Nursing Care,* by Ruth Stryker. W.B. Saunders Co., Philadelphia, Pennsylvania, 1972.
11. Community Health Services, Community Health Council of the United Community Fund of San Francisco, April 1960, p. 6.
12. *Handbook of Physical Medicine and Rehabilitation,* 2nd edition, by Frank Kruzen and F.V. Kottke. W.B. Saunders Co., Philadephia, Pennsylvania, 1972.
13. *Elements of Rehabilitation in Nursing,* by Rose Marie Boroch. C.V. Mosby Co.,

1976.

14. The Hospital as a Therapeutic Institution, *Bulletin of the Menninger Clinic,* *x:*66-70, 1946.

15. National Council on Rehabilitation, Symposium on the Process of Rehabilitation, Cleveland, Ohio, 1944.

16. Guidelines for Practice of Nursing in the Rehabilitative Team, American Nurses Association, New York, 1965.

17. An Experiment in the Rehabilitation of Nursing Home Residents, by H.R. Kelman. *Journal of Public Health, 77:*355-33, 1965.

18. Rehabilitation: A New Emphasis in Nursing Home Care, by H. Anderson. *Journal on Rehabilitation, 4:*30-33, 1965.

19. *Basic Rehabilitation Techniques,* by R.S. Sine, J.D. Holcomb, R.E. Rough, and S.E. Liss. Aspen Systems Corp., Century Blvd., Germantown, Maryland, 1977.

20. Rehabilitation and the Aged, by Lester E. Wolcott; Physiological and Biological Aspects of Aging, by Samuel Goldstein and William Reichel. In *Clinical Aspects of Aging,* by William Reichel. Williams & Wilkins, Baltimore, Maryland, 1978.

Chapter 7

REHABILITATION OF PATIENTS WITH SPECIFIC DISORDERS

INTRODUCTION TO NEUROLOGICAL DISABILITIES

IT is interesting to note that neurological disability affects 60 percent of the elderly patients, and of these 25 to 30 percent are long-term patients with hemiplegia. In most cases, a neurologic disability causes a functional impairment and is one of the most common causes of physical disability. For the staff workers to understand how they can help the patient in their care, they must have an understanding of the function of the nervous system. Many diseases and injuries cause neurological impairment; however, the impairment itself does not depend on the nature of the lesion but only on its site. For instance, if a certain area of the brain is damaged, the patient will develop spastic paralysis of the opposite side of the body. His disability and management will be the same regardless of the cause of this damage, which might have been a hemorrhage, a blood clot, a tumor, an abscess, or a bullet.

If it is a progressive disease, one must not only focus on the final state of the patients' rehabilitation but must strive for a status of functional ability that can be maintained according to their progress. If a patient with multiple sclerosis has paraplegia as his present disability, he should be at the same functional level as a patient whose paraplegia is a residual disability due to the spinal cord injury, but multiple sclerosis usually is progressive. It is advisable not to push a patient in his maximal performance because there must be some margin for neurologic deterioration without immediately changing the status and organization of the patient's environment, and without causing discouragement or despair.

PRINCIPLE CAUSES OF NEUROLOGIC IMPAIRMENT

Some degenerative, toxic, or infectious diseases selectively affect specific structures of the nervous system. For instance, epidemic encephalitis causes permanent damage to the basal ganglia only and may eventually lead to postencephalitic parkinsonism. Acute anterior poliomyelitis selectively attacks anterior horn cells in the gray matter of the cord leading to lower motor neuron flaccid paralysis. Some diseases may attack two structures selectively. For instance, the deficiency disease that causes pernicious anemia may cause, simultaneously, degeneration of the corticospinal tract and the fibers of the posterior column of the spinal cord. Transection of the spinal cord may be injury or invasion of the cord or brain by tumor and may result in multiple neurological impairments.

The brain and the spinal cord may be damaged by injuries, neoplasms, various infectious diseases, and deprivation of oxygen by cerebral vascular accidents, resulting in multiple neurological impairments.

CAUSES OF INCOORDINATION

The cerebellum and its pathways are responsible for coordination of movement and for equilibrium by way of connections with the vestibular system. It can be affected by the same lesions that damage the cerebral hemispheres, resulting in incoordination of voluntary motion and loss of balance, depending upon the site of the lesion. Proprioceptive nerve fibers can be involved in cerebellar disorders. Incoordination of the lower extremities is disabling, leading to an unsteady gait called ataxia.

Different Forms of Ataxia

1. Lower extremity ataxia interferes with locomotion.
2. Spinal ataxia is connected with a peculiar gait. The patient raises his legs higher than necessary and throws them out with greater force.

The lack of motor control actually is due to impaired or absent position sense. Improvement can be achieved by telling patients to keep their eyes fixed on their lower extremities. Also, climbing stairs will improve ataxia.

Definition of Incoordination

Incoordination is a disturbance of motor function in which smoothness and precision of motor are disturbed. Normal smoothness and precision of motion depends on extremely sensitive coordination of many muscle groups. Motor coordination requires and is regulated by constant sensory feedback of many data concerning tension in muscles, position of joints, and the position of the body and the limbs in relationship to each other and to gravity. The data is derived from the vestibular apparatus of the inner ear and from the retina, as well as from the proprioceptive sensory connections with joints and muscles.

Coordinated motion may be altered by many factors:

1. Muscle paralysis
2. Joint disturbances
3. Pain
4. Involuntary movements

The term ataxia is used frequently in the area of incoordination, since it is a disturbance of the proprioceptive impulses monitored by the cerebellum.

REHABILITATION OF THE PATIENT
WITH INCOORDINATION

Upper Extremity Involvement

The patient is greatly handicapped in all activities of daily living. If the ataxia (incoordination) is severe, the patient may need assistance with some of the activities of daily living. Usually they can do the activities of daily living, but it takes them much longer. They may get frustrated because they must try to do it two or three times before they are successful. Self-feeding can lead to food all over face, hands, table, and floor.

Some simple measures to improve hand activities and self-care activities are the following:

1. Proper stabilization of the trunk, usually the elbow.
2. Use of adapted equipment such as suction cups, food guards, special drinking cups with spouts to prevent spilling.

3. If ataxia is severe, it might be necessary to attach a weight to the upper extremity or restrict motion by braces that allow movement in only one direction.

4. In some cases, medication is indicated to relax the muscle and relieve nervous tension.

CAUSES OF INVOLUNTARY MOVEMENTS

Involuntary rhythmic, writhing, or twisting motions are due to pathology of the basal ganglia of the brain. Huntington's chorea is hereditary. St. Vitus's dance is an aftermath of rheumatic fever. Athetosis, a peculiar writhing motion, is frequently caused by damage due to lack of oxygen during childbirth. Parkinson's chorea, characterized by constant tremor and rigidity of the trunk and limbs may follow encephalitis or carbon monoxide poisoning or be due to arteriosclerosis. It is frequently seen in the elderly.

It is easy to understand that involuntary movements imply movements of the head, the trunk, or the extremities occurring spontaneously and purposelessly. The most common types of involuntary movements are the rhythmic motions of a segment of the body. In Parkinson's syndrome, they occur as tremors at rest, or they may occur on voluntary motion.

REHABILITATION OF INVOLUNTARY MOVEMENTS

Parkinson's Disease

Parkinson's disease is a common disease among many patients in nursing homes. Parkinson's disease is a sydrome caused by damage to the basal ganglia and occurs after epidemic encephalitis or diminished blood supply to the brain due to arteriosclerosis. It usually starts out as a shaking palsy at rest, but as it progresses, the tremors occur on any motion of any extremity. Further progression is muscular rigidity. Sometimes, patients develop a disturbance in their standing and ambulatory balance.

At present, the only program is one of delaying the progression of the disease by the use of —

1. range of motion exercises, daily;

2. assistance in ambulation.

Once patients rely on a wheelchair, their disease gets progressively worse, and they develop contractures and bed sores, which make their problems very serious. The key point in their rehabilitation is *activity*.

CAUSES OF LOWER MOTOR NEURON PARALYSIS

Lower motor neuron paralysis is the result of damage to the anterior horn cells in the gray matter of the cord or to their axons, which carry impulses to the voluntary muscle fibers. The damage may be caused by injury, occlusion of the anterior spinal artery, tumor, herniation of intervertebral disc, growth of bony spurs into the intervertebral foramina (spondylosis), chronic inflammation of the meninges, and anterior poliomyelitis.

CAUSES OF UPPER MOTOR NEURON PARALYSIS

1. Cerebral vascular accident — thrombus, embolus, rupture of a blood vessel. The latter is the most common in the elderly. Arteriosclerosis is a predisposing factor.
2. Tumor, abscess.
3. Selective degeneration.
4. Injury.
5. Transverse lesions of the spinal cord.

The most common neurological impairment is spastic paralysis. Upper motor neuron paralysis is classified according to the site of the paralysis. There are three types (Fig. 7-1).

Hemiplegia

A lesion in the motor cortex (area 4) and the premotor cortex (area 6) of one cerebral hemisphere will cause spastic paralysis on the opposite side of the body, which includes muscles of the head supplied by cranial nerves.

A lesion of the cervical spinal cord may cause hemiplegia on the same side if it involves only half of the cord. However, it usually involves both sides of the body, since the diameter of the cord is small and lesions are most often complete transverse ones.

A   *B*   *C*

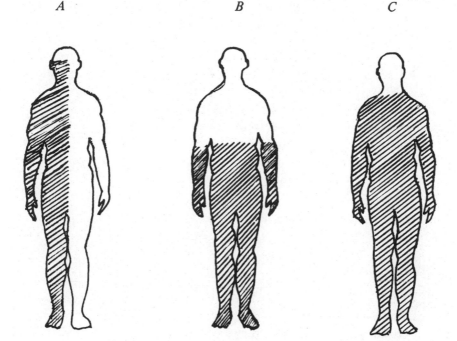

Figure 7-1. Illustration of the three types of paralysis. A. Hemiplegic. B. Paraplegic. C. Quadriplegic.

Concomitant damage to the adjacent sensory area (1,2,3) of the cerebral cortex will result in loss of sensation on the opposite side of the body, which adds to the disability.

Aphasia will be present if the lesion is on the dominant side.

Paraplegia

A complete transverse lesion of the spinal cord in the thoracic and upper lumbar regions will cause spastic paralysis of both lower extremities, but the upper extremities will be spared. The trunk musculature will be involved below the site of the lesion.

Quadriplegia

A transection of the spinal cord in the low cervical region will cause paralysis of all muscles below the lesion, all four extremities, and the trunk. If the lesion is in the brain stem, it may create bilateral involvement, but since the descending pyramidal tract is wider than the cord, unilateral involvement is a possibility. Brain stem and high cervical lesions cause paralysis of the intercostal muscles and the diaphram, which are the muscles of respiration. The victim usually dies in a very short time. The spinal cord proper terminates at the second lumbar vertebra. Below lumbar 2, in the vertebral foramen there are only spinal nerves lumbar 3, 4, 5 and the five sacral nerves, which carry lower motor neurons and sensory fibers. A lesion below lumbar 2 will cause flaccid paralysis of the lower extremities primarily, with loss of sensation.

GOALS FOR PATIENTS WITH HEMIPLEGIA, PARAPLEGIA, AND QUADRIPLEGIA

Hemiplegia

Patients with complete residual hemiplegia will become ambulatory and self-caring unless prevented from doing so by secondary disabilities. Most often they will be required to wear a short leg brace with a 90-degree plantar flexion stop, or if knee flexion is a problem, a long leg brace. Frequently hemiplegic patients use a cane. They usually become able to use public transportation as well as to drive a car.

Paraplegia

The paraplegic patient becomes self-caring and independent in the wheelchair. Some paraplegic patients may also become ambulatory with long leg braces and crutches. Paraplegic patients need specially modified automobiles for transportation if travel is to be independent.

Quadriplegia

Unless the involvement of the upper extremities is minimal, the quadriplegic requires an attendant. Whatever activity he is capable of carrying out for himself depends on the degree of involvement of the upper extremities. Usually, the typical quadriplegic whose disability is caused by transection of the lower cervical spinal cord can do the following: feed himself, write, wash his face and upper body, and wheel his chair. He usually needs some help in dressing and with transfer to and from the wheelchair.

We will go into more detail concerning the hemiplegic patient, since this condition is more prevalent in the nursing home than paraplegia and quadriplegia. In fact, the latter types very rarely are patients in nursing homes.

The Hemiplegic in Nursing Homes

Hemiplegic patients may have a right or left paralysis of the body. The cranial nerve involvement may be on the same side or on the opposite side of that of the trunk and extremities. If no voluntary motion is possible on the hemiplegic side, the hemiplegia is complete; if some voluntary motion is present, the hemiplegia is partial (hemiparesis). Frequently, hemiplegia is associated with additional neurological disabilities, i.e. aphasia. The upper motor neuron hemiplegia, sometimes called a stroke, is usually a lesion in one cerebral hemisphere.

WHAT IS THE PROGNOSIS FOR THE FUTURE? If complete recovery occurs, it is accomplished usually within two months. These cases are called transient hemiplegia. If complete recovery does not occur, the patient is left with a residual hemiplegia that may be complete or incomplete. In addition to paralysis, sensory defects may, and frequently do, add to the residual disability. If there is progression of neurologic abnormality and increasing spasticity, usually an expanding lesion or additional cerebral vascular disorder is responsible.

WHAT FUNCTIONAL IMPROVEMENTS CAN BE EXPECTED? If the hemiplegia is the only disability, the patient with complete residual hemiplegia can become ambulatory and self-caring within four weeks. He may have to wear a short or long leg brace and possibly walk with a cane for a period of time. If additional disabilities are present, the prognosis covers a wide spectrum of functional levels ranging from complete self-care to full dependence on nursing care.

WHAT ARE THE GOALS? They should be —

1. achievement of mobility and ambulation;
2. achievement of self-care;

3. psychosocial adjustment to disability;
4. prevention of secondary disabilities.

HOW ARE THE GOALS ACHIEVED? Delay in achieving mobility and ambulation is often due to the mistaken opinion that these functions can be restored only after some motion returns to the paralyzed limbs. It is most important, as a basic principle of rehabilitation, to work with what the patient has. In hemiplegia, this is the uninvolved half of the body as well as the involved. Even if there is no return of voluntary function in the paralyzed limbs, the hemiplegic patient is potentially capable of moving about in bed, transferring from bed to chair and to wheelchair to toilet, and ambulating independently. It is surprising, but moving about in bed requires greater strength and effort than transfer and ambulation.

To facilitate moving in bed with safety, the patient needs side rails and an overhead trapeze for support. Transfer from bed to chair or from bed to commode by teaching patients to put their weight on their good leg and to use their uninvolved arm for balance and support are easy goals.

There are four phases to the restoration of mobility and ambulation:

1. A non-weight bearing phase or bed phase.
2. A unilateral weight bearing or stand up phase.
3. Bilateral weight-bearing phase.
4. Stair climbing and cane walking.

Activities for Phase One — Bed Phase

In the hemiplegic patient without other complications, the time for a patient to be bedfast will usually be one to three days. In complicated cases, there is no definite period for this bed phase.

The bed must be firm and smooth so that patients do not sink into a hole. One should be able to slide body and extremities from side to side. There should be a footboard so that they can move legs freely and prevent footdrop. Side rails should be placed for safety and to use for movements, and a trapeze for the use of the uninvolved hand is also necessary.

One must understand that the patient immediately after a stroke may be entirely helpless. It is important to reassure him that some function will return on the hemiplegic side, but the staff must point out that it is most important to strengthen the uninvolved side. Quite often, patients will rebel at the thought that nothing is being done for the hemiplegic side and resent exercises prescribed for the uninvolved side. Thus, the pathology of this problem must be explained in simple terms, indicating the possibility of some return of voluntary function within a short time. Regardless of return, it must be pointed out that if he makes the maximum effort to recover in three to four weeks he may be back to some degree of normalcy. Exercising the uninvolved side indirectly helps the involved side. Patients must be told that gradual strengthening of the uninvolved side will parallel progress from bed, to standing, and then to walking. The role of reflex function and the purpose of the leg brace must be explained. The schedule of exercises should be discussed, letting the patient give you his ideas on exercises. Explain how his mobility and ambulation will be integrated into other phases of rehabilitation and with his daily activities, such as eating, voiding, defecating, bathing, dressing, exercising, entertaining of visitors, resting, and his recreating.

The purpose of bed exercises for the stroke patient are as follows:

1. To strengthen the uninvolved side
2. To enable the patient to change positions in bed
3. To prepare him for increasing self-care
4. To achieve transfer ability

The bed exercises are very strenuous for the acute hemiplegic patient if they are initated after the stroke. Futhermore, they are strenuous because of the difficulty of moving one's body in bed with the use of only one leg and one arm. Therefore, the exercise period must be brief. In order to achieve some strengthening with brief exercise periods, patients must exercise frequently. It is important also to progress gradually from the easiest bed exercises to the strenuous ones as the patient's strength increases.

It is most important that during the bed phase the patient should take precautions to prevent secondary disabilities by the following:

1. Proper positioning of all extremities, particularly the shoulder.
2. Range of motion exercises to prevent atrophy and contractures.
3. Simple self-care activities may be performed such as feeding,

bathing, use of urinal, writing.

Stand-Up Phase

The stand-up phase starts as soon as patients have acquired the ability to move themselves unassisted into a sitting position on the edge of the bed. At this time patients will get braces, if needed. A heavy high-backed armchair that is stable is necessary equipment. The main objectives of the stand-up phase is to develop —

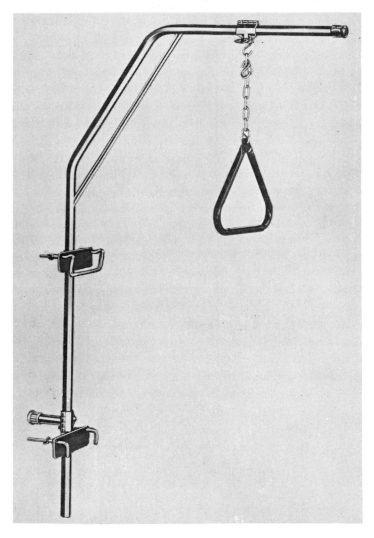

Figure 7-2. End of bed trapeze.

1. strength in the trunk;
2. strength and dexterity in the uninvolved lower extremity;
3. standing balance.

The patient must use his uninvolved leg rather than his arm to pull himself upright from the bed. Once the patient is standing, he must try to develop stability and balance endurance. To develop balance, he should try to exercise by leaning to the left and then to the right. *Caution:* Patients tire easily. Each session should be short and held at least four to six times a day. One method that can be used would be for the patient to stand after each mealtime, plus getting into a chair to eat. If the patient complains about fatigue, watch him. Do not push, just encourage him. Point out that the more he

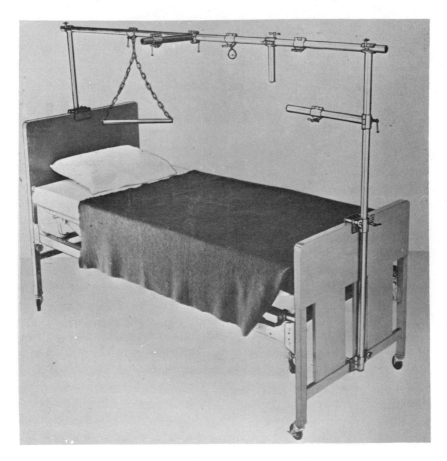

Figure 7-3. Trapeze over entire bed.

does, the faster he will be able to walk. Do not help patients; each time they accomplish something by themselves, their morale is helped. If the staff helps them, it reminds them that they have a disability, thus retarding their rehabilitation.

The preceding program is carried out until the patient has mastered the standing technique, can arise with ease from a chair to standard height, and has the strength and balance, plus the endurance, needed for gait training. Figures 7-2, 7-3, and 7-4 show some exercise equipment and its use.

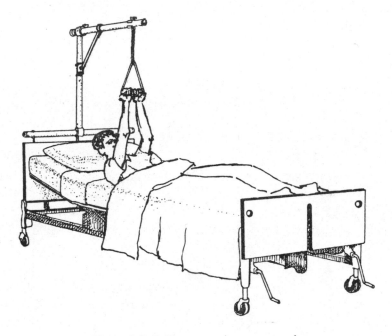

Figure 7-4. Pulling up, using a trapeze bar.

Exercises should be done three or four times a day when the patient is well rested. If exercises are done correctly, the patient should gain strength daily.

Groups of Exercises

1. Bed Phase

   a. Beginning Exercises

      (1) Turn over to the paralyzed side by grasping the side rail (Fig. 7-5).

(2) Turn over to the uninvolved side by grasping a low side rail or the mattress edge.

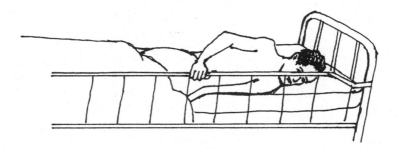

Figure 7-5. Beginning exercise of bed phase. Turn over to the paralyzed side by grasping the side rail.

(3) Pull up into half-sitting or full-sitting position by grasping the trapeze bar (Fig. 7-6).

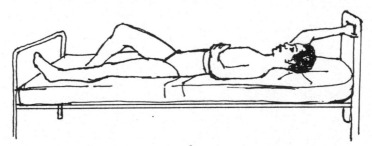

Figure 7-6. Intermediate exercise of bed phase. Pull the paralyzed leg toward the edge of the bed with the uninvolved leg, which has been slipped under it. The same position can be used for exercise in sliding up and down the bed by grasping the bar at the end of the bed and helping with the neck and the uninvolved leg.

b. Intermediate Exercises
  (1) Turn to either side beyond an angle of 90 degrees.
  (2) Slide up and down in bed grasping the bar at the head of the bed and helping with the neck and the uninvolved leg.
  (3) Pull the paralyzed leg toward the edge of the bed with the uninvolved leg, which has been slipped under it (Fig. 7-7).

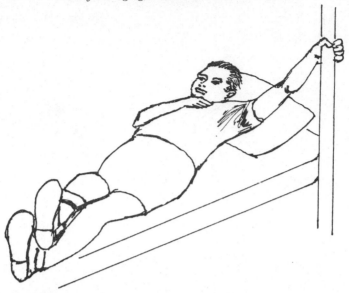

Figure 7-7. Intermediate exercise of bed phase. Moving legs over to the side of the bed. The involved leg is carried by the uninvolved leg.

c. Advanced Exercises
  (1) Slide sideways in bed grasping side rail. The moving is done with the use of leg, neck, and shoulder.

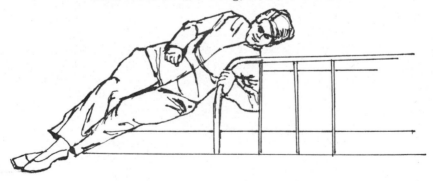

Figure 7-8. Bed phase exercise. Pull up into a half-sitting or full-sitting position by grasping the side rail. This exercise can also be used to teach transfer. The patient supports the weak arm across this chest and the weak leg with the stronger one. He then turns fully onto the side, pulling himself up with his strong arm as his legs go over the edge of the bed.

(2) Sit up on the edge of the bed, after lifting the paralyzed leg over the edge of the bed (Fig. 7-8).

Technique for Transfer

If the patient has learned how to stand and balance himself, he is ready to learn how to transfer from bed to a chair or wheelchair. The technique is simple: Stand up and pivot on the uninvolved leg and sit down in a chair. The arm of the chair can be used to balance while pivoting (Fig. 7-9). When patients become able to stand up from the bed and get into a chair, this gives them a tremendous boost to their morale. They can then use a commode, can eat in a

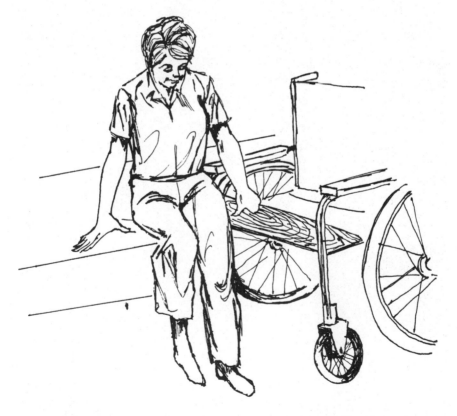

Figure 7-9. Transfer. Transferring from bed to wheelchair. The patient maintains balance by keeping his trunk a little forward and supporting his trunk with his arms by placing his hands in front of his hips to achieve a tripod position.

chair, and can move around, which makes them mobile.

TRANSFERS

As soon as the patient can sit alone on the side of his bed, he is ready to learn to transfer. In most cases it should *not* be necessary to *lift* the hemiplegic patient from bed to wheelchair and back onto the toilet, etc. Most patients can learn to transfer easily and safely without assistance. Initially, some physical and appropriate verbal support may be needed. Supervision should be given until the patient can transfer with security and confidence. Be sure that the patient wears shoes.

The principles that follow are applicable to most transfers other than the high bed.

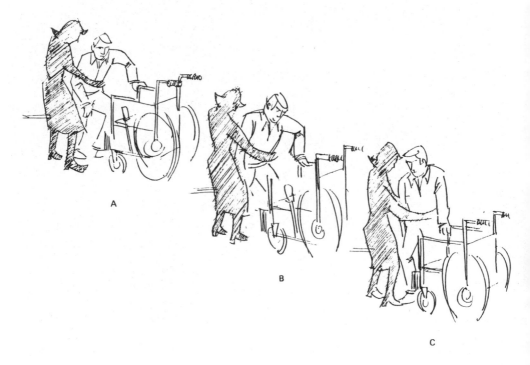

Figure 7-10. A. Wheelchair in place at the foot of patient's bed, with brakes locked, ready for transfer. B. Helper faces patient and prepares to brace the patient's weak knee with his knee. C. Standing up.

Transfers are made toward the patient's unaffected side. The chair is placed parallel to or at a slight angle to the bed on the unaffected side, facing the foot of the bed. If a wheelchair is used, it must have brakes, and they must be locked.

If assistance is needed a secure belt, "transfer belt," around the patient's waist should be used to provide a firm hand hold. The helper should stand facing the patient at a point where he can, if necessary, brace the patient's weak knee with his knee.

To stand up, the patient is instructed to slide to the edge of the bed and pull his feet well back under him. The patient grasps the nearest arm of the chair or places his good hand on the bed beside him, bends well forward, and pushes himself to a standing position. If assistance is needed at first it can be given by means of the transfer belt to provide a firm grip (Fig. 7-10).

After a *pause* in the standing position so that the patient can gain his balance, he should shift his good hand to the other arm of the chair and pivot until his back is to the chair. (Fig. 7-11).

The patient then sits down in a controlled manner, again bending forward at the waist as he does so (Fig. 7-12).

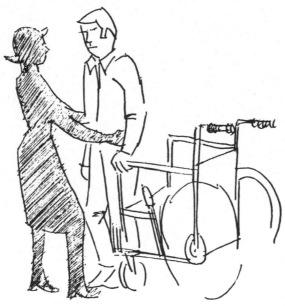

Figure 7-11. Pivoting from the standing position until back faces the chair.

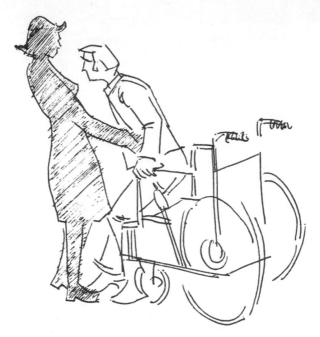

Figure 7-12. Sitting in a controlled manner.

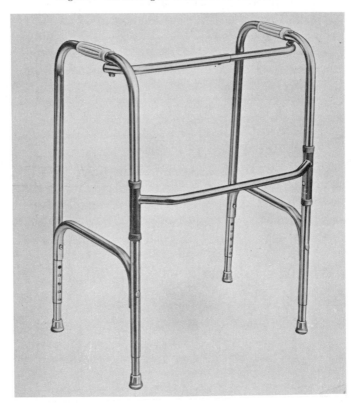

Figure 7-13. Standard walker.

AMBULATION

As soon as patients have gained strength, they can use a walker. They should be given proper training in the handling of a four-legged walker. They should use the walker only for short distances (20 feet) until they learn to use it properly. Figures 7-13, 7-14, and 7-15 show some common walkers.

Use of Steps

Steps are used as a total rehabilitative measure for patients to develop their total potential strength. During this activity, they use their lower extremities, trunk, arms, and shoulders. Usually, the

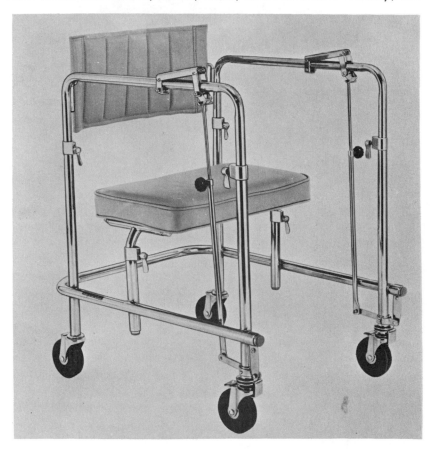

Figure 7-14. Walker with casters and a seat.

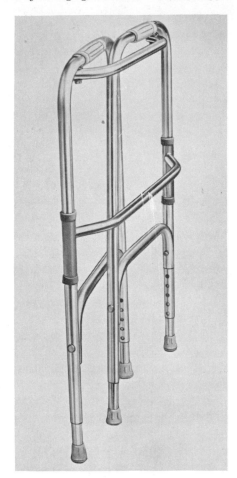

Figure 7-15. Folding walker.

steps are not undertaken for at least three to four weeks after the operation. It is suggested that patients start with 2-inch steps and gradually build up until they can walk up and down regular-size steps. First, the patient starts using the uninvolved leg to climb up the steps then down the steps the same way. Later, he can lead off with the involved leg in climbing steps.

The patient is now able to go to the physical therapy room for stair climbing training.

Suggestions for the steps:

1. Steps width should be greater than shoe length.
2. There should be overhang for a shoe to catch on.

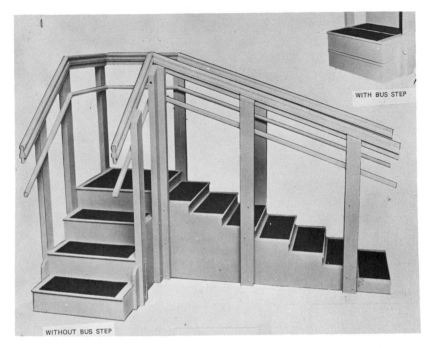

WITH BUS STEP

WITHOUT BUS STEP

Figure 7-16. Stairs.

3. Height of steps should vary from normal to deep to shallow.

How to Make Steps

Steps are made out of wood, six steps, 4 inches high, 36 inches wide. Platform is 24 inches by 36 inches.

Four steps are 6-inch steps. Overall size is 24 inches by 36 inches. First railing is 29 inches from floor; second railing is 31 inches from floor.

The advantages of stair climbing before gait training is that the psychological effect of the rise of the steps gives the patient the impression or sensation of being less far from the ground and of blocking his fall. If stair climbing is done with the added safety of the hand on the railing, there is much less hazard than is involved in walking on level ground. Other advantages are the following:

1. Climbing steps has greater exercise value than normal walking.
2. Patients learn to lift their feet, to flex hips and knees.

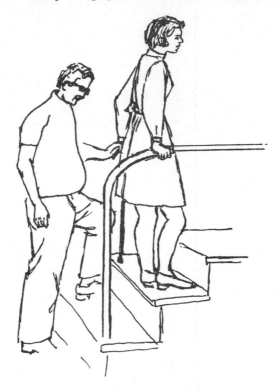

Figure 7-17. Stair climbing and descending. Climbing steps: Place hand on rail ahead of body. Lift uninvolved foot to first step. Step up. Bring the involved leg up beside the uninvolved leg. Repeat procedure. Always lead with the uninvolved leg. Descending steps: Place hands on rail ahead of body. Lift involved leg and step down one step; descend slowly, keeping control with the uninvolved leg. Bring the uninvolved leg beside the involved leg. Repeat until the patient reaches the floor.

 3. Patients begin to lead with the uninvolved leg.
 4. Patients can raise body with the uninvolved leg.
 5. Patients learn to take small, even steps.
 6. It influences coordination and control of the body.
 7. It strengthens the uninvolved side.

Techniques for stair climbing consist of two phases (Fig. 7-17):

 1. Going up the steps
  a. Place hand on rail ahead of body, over center of first step.
  b. Step up with the uninvolved foot.
  c. Place the involved foot next to it.

    d. Move hand upward on rail.

    e. Repeat, repeat, repeat.

This first phase is difficult because patients do not have trust or faith that the uninvolved leg will support them while they raise up to the next level.

  2. Going Down Stairs

    a. Stand with both feet on the top step, with hand on rail at the side.

    b. Step down with the involved foot.

    c. Bring uninvolved foot down beside the involved foot.

    d. Move hand downward on rail.

    e. Repeat until patient reaches the floor.

Cane Walking

The purpose of the cane is to take the place of the rail that was used for climbing steps. Some people do not need any training; they are able to make their own adjustment and ambulate accordingly. The cane is for stability and is to be used as such. Figures 7-18 through 7-25 show different types of canes and their use in climbing stairs and walking.

Cane Gaits

Three-point gait:

1. Advance uninvolved hand with cane until cane tip is one shoe length ahead of toes and about 6 to 8 inches out to the side. Push on cane, keeping body upright.
2. Advance involved foot one shoe length, heel even with the uninvolved toe; shift weight to involved foot and cane held by uninvolved hand.
3. Advance uninvolved foot through to one shoe length ahead of foot involved.
4. Repeat, repeat, repeat.

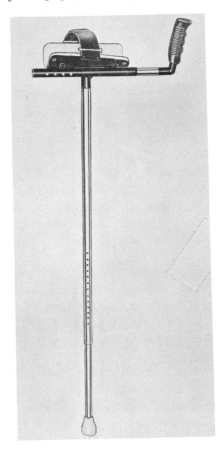

Figure 7-18. Forearm cane.

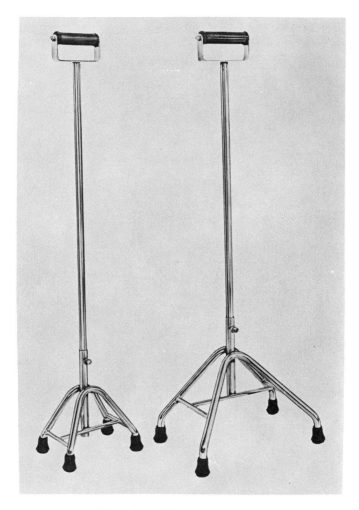

Figure 7-19. Four-pointed cane.

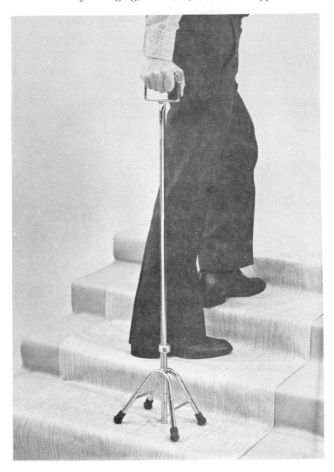

Figure 7-20. Using the four-pointed cane to climb stairs.

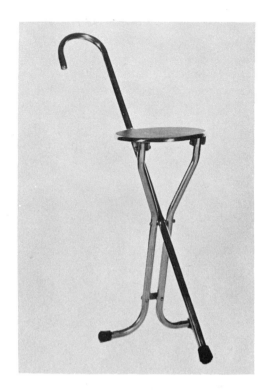

Figure 7-21. Cane with table rest.

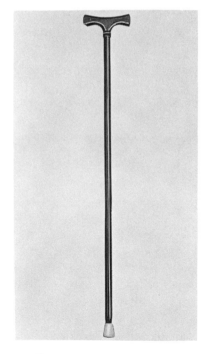

Figure 7-22. Straight cane.

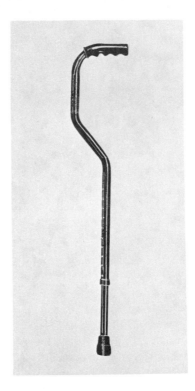

Figure 7-23. Curved cane.

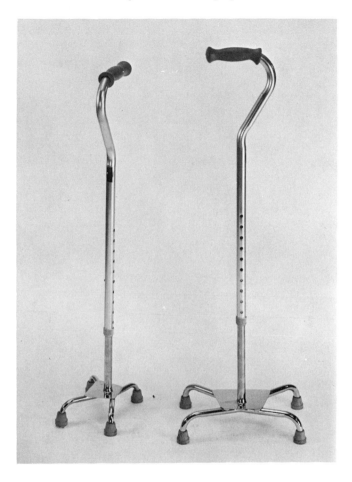

Figure 7-24. Another style of four-pointed cane.

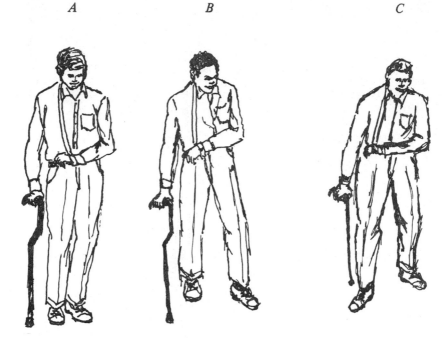

Figure 7-25. Standing with cane. A. Patient stands with cane on the strong side. B. Patient moves the cane and the weak leg ahead together. C. Patient then brings his strong leg forward.

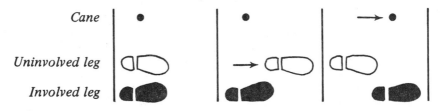

Figure 7-26. Three-point gait.

Two-point gait:
1. With weight on the involved foot and the cane, advance uninvolved foot one shoe length to bring heel even with the toes of the involved foot.
2. With all weight on the uninvolved foot, cane and involved foot move from the ground simultaneously and advance one shoe length beyond the uninvolved foot.

3. Repeat, repeat.

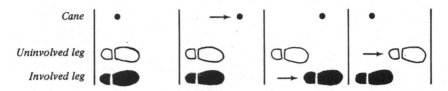

Figure 7-27. Two-point gait.

The different gaits are illustrated because people are different. Some can readily learn the two-point gait in which the cane is brought forward at the same time and the same distance as the involved foot.

DAILY LIVING ACTIVITIES

Self-Care

Restoration of self-care after a person has become mobile is the next important step in the rehabilitation of the hemiplegic patient. The loss of the function of one arm and one leg should not deter the person who wants to be independent from achieving his aims and goals.

Eating Activities

In the early stages of his recovery, the patient may need assistance in eating, but as soon as possible he should be encouraged to feed himself using his unaffected hand. Self-feeding can be started as soon as the patient can sit up in bed.

SUGGESTIONS FOR DEPENDENT FEEDING

1. With the patient's head turned toward his unaffected side, place the food in the unaffected side of his mouth.

2. If there is considerable involvement, place one hand on the cheek of the affected side to facilitate swallowing.

3. After each feeding check the cheek on the affected side for lodged food, which may be aspirated and choke the patient.

4. Because of the difficulty in chewing, the patient may have to chop his food or put it through a blender. As soon as possible, the

patient should have normal food. Careful evaluation of the diet may indicate the need for food supplements, which can be recommended by the patient's physician.

SUGGESTIONS FOR INDEPENDENT FEEDING

1. Initially it may be necessary to guide the patient's hand in holding the spoon, putting the food on the spoon, and bringing the food to his mouth. Have the patient feed himself part of the meal, observing him for signs of fatigue. As the patient improves, gradually increase independence in eating and encourage dining with other people.

2. Problems involved in one-handed eating may be overcome by using simple equipment. Certain adaptations such as a bread holder and food guard may be needed immediately. As the patient gains skill, this special equipment may no longer be necessary. Figures 7-28 through 7-34 show utensils adapted for use by the handicapped patient.

a. A suction cup, rubber mat, or wet cloth may be placed under the plate to keep it stationary.

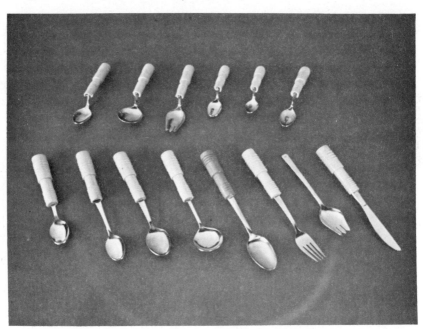

Figure 7-28. Odd-shaped utensils used for the handicapped.

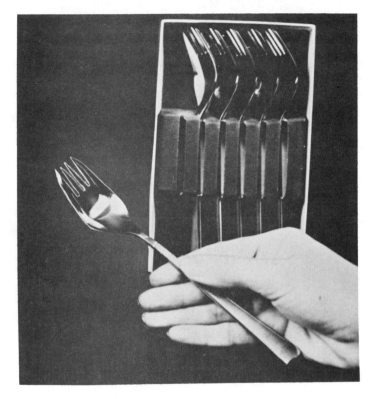

Figure 7-29. Four-pronged fork.

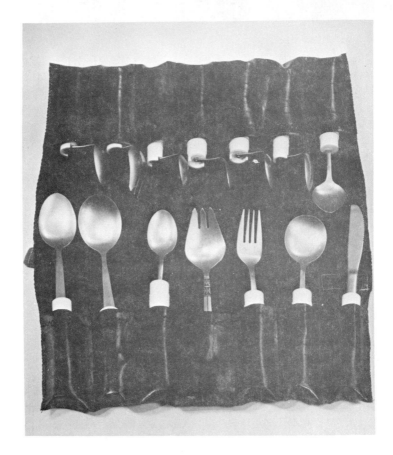

Figure 7-30. Different types of utensils.

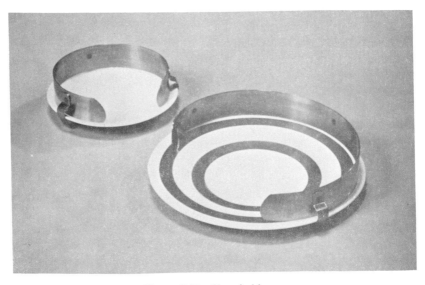

Figure 7-31. Plate holder.

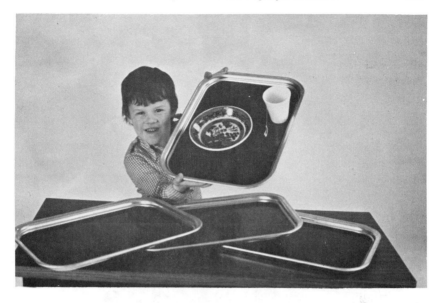

Figure 7-32. Tray that does not allow plate to slide.

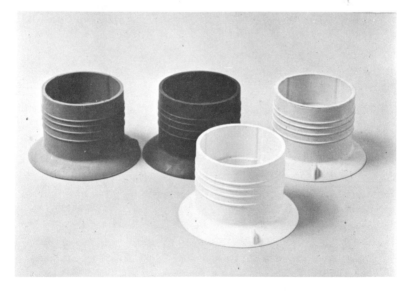

Figure 7-33. Holders for glasses. These could also be used for soup.

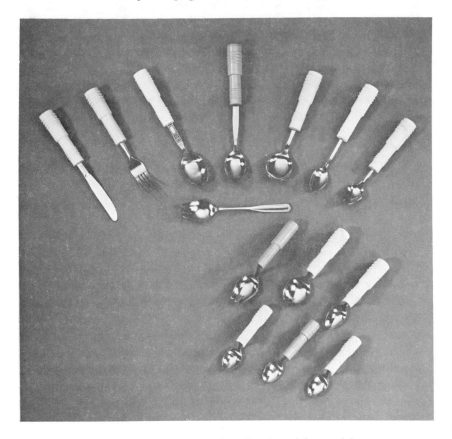

Figure 7-34. Another set of utensils adapted for special use.

b. To keep a drinking straw stationary, the straw may be secured with cellophane tape or placed through a hole in a paper cover over the glass. Plastic tubing sometimes is easier for the patient to use, as it does not collapse as easily as a paper straw. Straw drinking should be replaced by a cup or glass as soon as the patient is able to use one of them.

c. A food guard may be used to prevent food from sliding off the plate.

d. A rocking knife or sharp steak knife may be used to enable a patient to cut his own food. One-handled cutting is done by rocking the knife back and forth rather than cutting in the conventional way.

e. To butter bread, press the knife down as the soft butter is drawn across the bread, or place the thumb on the bread and pull the knife toward it. A bread holder made from a 4-inch square board with nails in the corners is helpful.

f. If the patient has visual difficulty, it may be necessary to call his attention to food on each side of his plate.

Bathing

The patient may begin independent bathing activities early in his convalescence. While still a bed patient, he may begin washing his own face and hands and ultimately progress to independent bed bathing. When the patient can transfer to a wheelchair, he may be taught how to take a tub bath or shower while seated on a bench or a chair.

SUGGESTIONS FOR BATHING

1. A sponge is easier to use than a washcloth, particularly while the patient is still in bed. If a washcloth is used, it can be folded in half and sewed on two sides to make a mitt.

2. A brush with a suction cup will enable the patient to clean the unaffected hand. To wash the unaffected arm, place a cloth or mitt in or around the affected hand and move the unaffected arm over or under it.

3. A long-handled bath sponge with a place in the sponge for soap will help the patient reach most parts of his body.

4. A shower spray on a hose can be used while the patient is seated on a chair in the tub. Disconnect the hose immediately following completion of the bath. (*Note:* If a permanent shower spray is connected to the tub faucet, a plumber should install the fixture in a manner that will prevent bath water from gaining entrance into the water line.)

5. Hand rails, removable grab bars, and safety tread tape will help insure the patient's safety.

PROCEDURE FOR TUB BATHING

When the patient has good standing balance, muscle strength, and sufficient joint mobility, he is ready to attempt tub bathing. Initially, the assistance of one person may be needed to support and stabilize the affected side. As the patient gains skill and confidence, less supervision will be needed.

1. Place a chair or bench with rubber crutch tips on the legs of a

friction surface, such as a towel or safety tread, in the tub.

2. Place another chair parallel to the tub so that the patient's affected side will be next to the tub.

3. The patient sits on the chair. While sitting, he picks up his affected leg and places it in the tub.

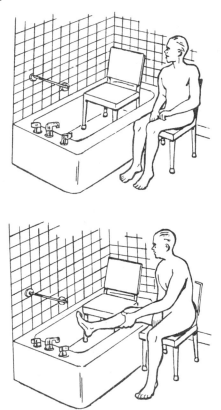

4. With his unaffected arm and leg he pushes himself from one chair to the chair in the tub.

5. While the patient is on the chair in the tub, he lifts the unaffected leg into the tub.

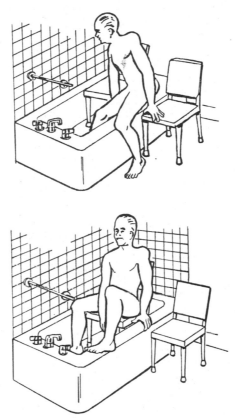

6. To get out of the tub, the procedure is reversed, with the patient moving toward the unaffected side.

7. The use of a transfer board will provide greater safety for some patients. The board, such as a table leaf, is placed on the chairs and the patient slides along the board from one chair to the other.

PROCEDURE FOR SHOWER BATH

Shower stalls are obviously more convenient for bathing, but safety precautions must still be observed. A chair placed in the shower for the patient to sit on makes bathing easier and safer. Large crutch tips can be put on all four chair legs to prevent the chair from slipping. Safety treads on the floor are a necessary safety measure.

Grooming

Grooming activities can also be started while the patient is still in bed. Hair combing, teeth brushing, shaving, and application of makeup can usually be accomplished with one hand if the patient is shown how. Only daily practice can perfect the skill.

SUGGESTIONS FOR GROOMING

1. A brush with a suction cup can be attached to the basin for cleaning dentures.

2. Toilet articles packaged in pressurized cans or plastic containers are easier and safer to use than screw-top glass containers.

3. Screw-top containers may be opened and closed by pressing the container on foam rubber or holding it between the knees.

4. Mirrors that clip around a knee or around the neck eliminate the need for holding the mirror or for standing to use the mirror.

5. By puffing out his cheeks or making faces, the patient can keep his skin taut while shaving. Electric shavers are easier to use than safety razors.

6. Hair combing is primarily a one-handed activity and can be done easily if the hair is kept at a reasonable length and in a simple style.

7. It is convenient to have articles such as nail files taped down.

Dressing

A patient should be taught to dress himself as soon as he can sit by himself. He may begin by dressing himself in sleeping attire, but this should soon be discarded for street clothes. At first he will require help in dressing so that he will not become too discouraged. With careful teaching, encouragement, and a few minor clothing adaptations, he can achieve independence in this activity.

The proper clothing is very essential to a hemiplegic. All clothing should be loose fitting and have wide sleeves and trouser legs. The buttons and zippers should be placed in front. If a person has a long or short leg brace, his trouser leg should be cut and a zipper inserted.

In putting on shirts, blouses, or coats, the involved arm should be placed first in sleeve (Fig. 7-35).

SUGGESTIONS FOR DRESSING

1. Clothing made of materials that do not wrinkle easily and that are easily laundered such as polyester, nylon, seersucker, or wrinkleshed cotton will prove most serviceable. Clothing a size larger than

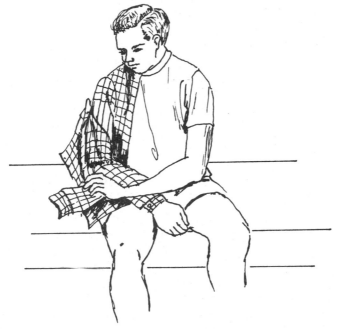

Figure 7-35. Upper extremity dressing. Putting on shirt — the patient applies sleeve to the weaker arm first. The remainder of the shirt can then be put behind him and brought around to the stronger arm.

usual will be easier to put on and take off.

2. For women, dresses that open down the front, have fairly wide arm holes, and have full skirts are more convenient. Brassieres that open in the front and half slips may be easier to manage.

3. For men, loose-fitting clothes are best. Pre-tied neckties solve a problem for those who have difficulty in tying with one hand. In tying a necktie with one hand, a clothespin to secure the narrow end of the tie to the shirt might make the procedure easier. Shirt sleeve buttons sewn with elastic thread can be kept buttoned, eliminating the need for assistance in buttoning.

4. Velcro® closures (two surfaces of nylon tape that adhere to each other securely when merely pressed together) may be more easily managed than zippers and are available at local department stores.

5. Elastic shoelaces, hooks, or zipper locks eliminate shoe tying.

6. When performing dressing activities, it is preferable for the patient to be seated in an armchair or in a wheelchair with the

brakes locked. If the patient has good sitting balance, a straight chair may be used. In either case, both feet should be on the floor.

FRONT-OPENING SHIRT

The following methods can be used for any garment that opens completely down the front such as a pajama top, a blouse, or a dress. The patient should be seated with his feet flat on the floor.

Procedure for Putting on a Front-opening Shirt — Method I

1. Grasp the collar and shake the shirt out with the unaffected hand. Place the shirt on the lap with the label toward the chest and facing up.

2. Position the sleeve for the affected arm so that the opening is as large and as close to the involved hand as possible.

3. Place the affected hand into the sleeve. Then pull the sleeve up over the elbow and under the armpit.

4. Put the unaffected arm into the other sleeve, then raise the arm and shake the sleeve into position past the elbow.

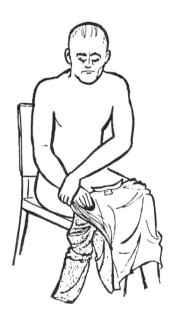

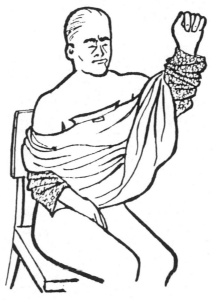

5. Gather the garment up the middle of the back from hem to collar with the unaffected hand, and raise the shirt over the head. Duck the head, then lean forward, passing the shirt over the head.

6. With the unaffected hand, work the shirt down past the shoulder on both sides. Reach to the back and pull the tail of the shirt down. Line up the shirt fronts for buttoning.

7. Begin buttoning with the bottom button, which is in full view.

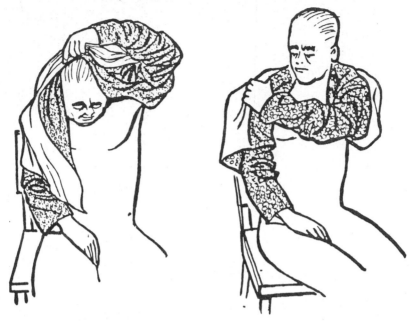

Procedure for Putting on a Front-opening Shirt — Method II

1. Place the affected arm in the proper sleeve and work the sleeve onto the arm and up over the shoulder.

2. Pull the material over the affected shoulder and around the back.

3. Slip the unaffected arm into the armhole.

4. Adjust the shirt and fasten the buttons.

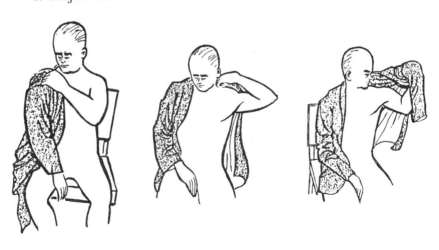

Procedure for Removing a Front-opening Shirt — Method I

1. Unbutton the garment.
2. Lean forward and free the garment in back.
3. With the unaffected arm gather the material up in back of the neck (or take hold of the collar). While leaning forward, duck the head and pull the garment over the head.
4. Remove the shirt from the unaffected arm first and then from the affected arm.

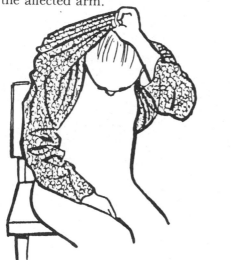 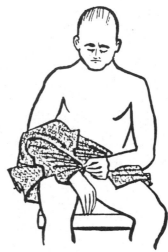

Procedure for Removing a Front-opening Shirt — Method II

1. Take the unaffected arm out of the shirt sleeve.
2. Remove the shirt from the back using the unaffected hand.
3. Remove the affected arm.

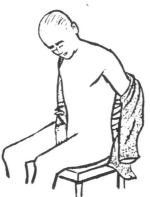 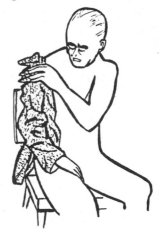

PULLOVER SHIRT

The following method can be used for any garment that goes over the head.

Procedure for Putting on a Pullover Shirt

1. Place the shirt on the lap with the bottom toward the chest and the label facing down.

2. With the unaffected hand, roll the bottom edge of the shirt up to the sleeve on the affected side.

3. Open the sleeve and place the affected arm into the proper opening. Then pull the shirt up the arm past the elbow.

4. Insert the unaffected arm into the remaining sleeve.

5. Adjust the shirt on the affected side up and onto the shoulder.

6. Gather the shirt back with the unaffected hand, lean forward, duck the head, then pass the shirt over the head.

7. Adjust the shirt.

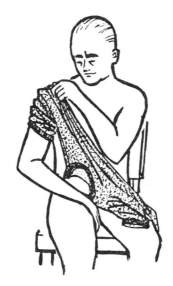

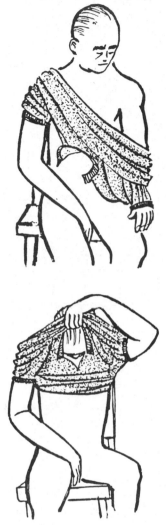

Procedure for Removing a Pullover Shirt

1. Starting at the top of the back, gather the shirt up, lean forward, duck the head, and pull the shirt forward over the head.

2. Remove the shirt from the unaffected arm first and then from the affected arm.

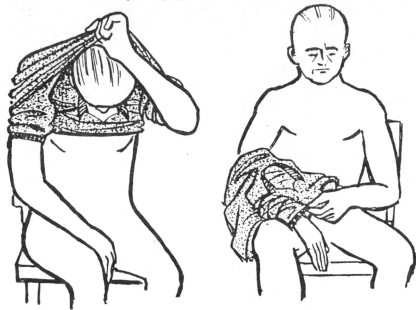

Trousers

Trousers, shorts, and panties must be put on in a lying or sitting position. First, the leg opening is pulled over the leg, then the uninvolved leg steps into the other opening. If the patient is lying on his back, he raises his buttocks off the bed by pushing down with his good leg, which is flexed at hip and knee, and at the same time pulls the trousers up to his waist (Fig. 7-36).

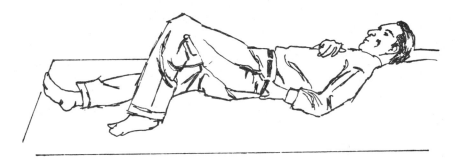

Figure 7-36. Lower extremity dressing. If the patient has left hemiplegia, he bends his left knee and raises his left hip. He then turns onto his left side to adjust the trousers on the right.

Procedure for Putting on Trousers in a Sitting Position

1. Sit in a straight arm chair or in a wheelchair.
2. Place the unaffected leg directly in front of the midline of the body with the knee flexed to 90 degrees. Using the unaffected hand, place the affected leg over the unaffected leg in a crossed-leg position.
3. Slip the trouser leg over the affected foot and pull it up to the knee. Do not pull the trousers above the knee.

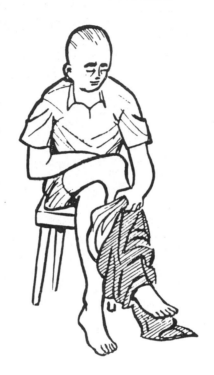

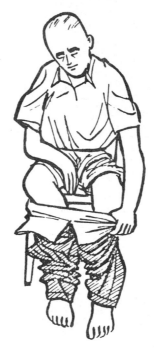

4. Uncross the affected leg.

5. Put the unaffected leg in the trousers and work the trousers onto the hips as far as possible. This can be done by sitting first on one hip and then on the other.

6. Now stand and pull the trousers up over the hips. To prevent the trousers from dropping during standing, place the affected hand into the pocket or use suspenders and pull them into position on the shoulder before standing.

7. To fasten the trousers, it is easier to fasten the belt while standing. The patient can sit or stand to fasten the fly.

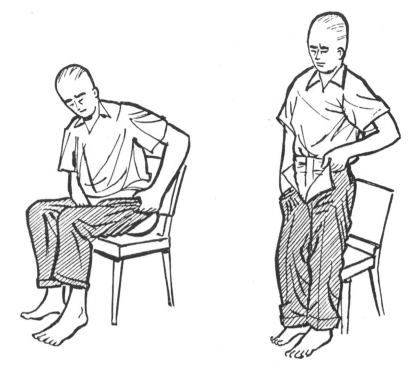

Procedure for Putting on Trousers Lying Down

In cases of poor balance, putting on and taking off trousers can best be done on the bed.

1. Place the affected leg in a bent position and cross it over the unaffected leg.

2. Straighten the trousers and work them onto the affected leg up to the knee. Uncross the leg.

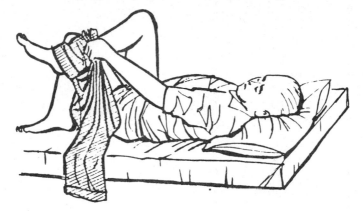

3. Insert the unaffected leg in the trousers and work them onto the hips as far as possible.

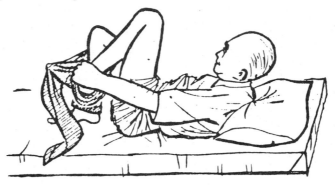

4. Work the trousers over the hips by rolling from side to side. Another method is to bend the good leg, press down with the foot and shoulder, elevate the hips from the bed, and then pull the trousers over the hips.

5. Fasten the trousers.

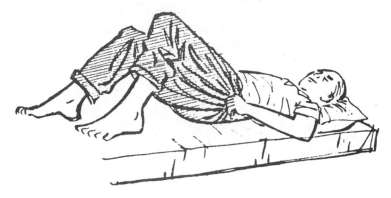

Procedure for Removing Trousers Sitting Up

1. While sitting, the patient unfastens the trousers and works them down past his hips as far as possible.

2. The patient stands and lets the trousers drop past his hips.

3. The patient sits and removes the unaffected leg from the trousers.

4. Then the patient crosses the affected leg over the unaffected leg, removes the trousers, and uncrosses the leg.

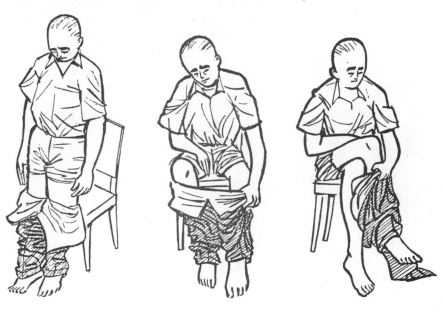

Procedure for Removing Trousers Lying Down

Refer to the diagrams for putting on trousers lying down.

1. Hike the hips as in putting on the trousers.

2. Work the trousers down past the hips and remove the unaffected leg first.

STOCKINGS

For putting on socks or stockings, the involved leg is picked up and crossed over the good leg so that the foot can be reached. Getting the shoes on can best be handled with a long-handled shoehorn. It is easiest to avoid using shoelaces altogether. Figures 7-37, 7-38, and 7-39 show useful tools for shoes and stockings.

The following method can be used for stockings or socks:

1. The patient sits with the unaffected leg directly in front of the midline of his body with the affected leg crossed over it.

2. He should roll the stocking to within several inches of the toe and open the stocking by putting the thumb and first two fingers into the stocking.

3. Place the rolled stocking over the toes of the foot, then the re-

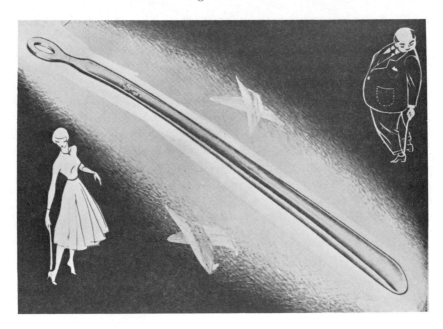

Figure 7-37. Long-handled shoehorn. Courtesy of J.A. Preston, New York.

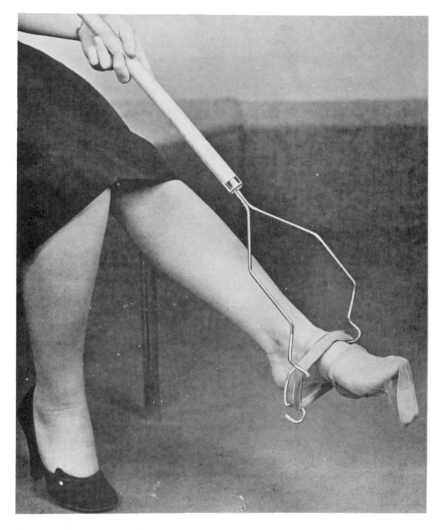

Figure 7-38. Long-handled instrument used to pull up hose. Courtesy of J.A. Preston, New York.

maining portion can be brought onto the leg without twisting it.

SHOES

The following method can be used for shoes with or without braces:

Procedure for Putting on Shoes with Short Leg Brace

1. Place the unaffected foot on the floor directly in front of the

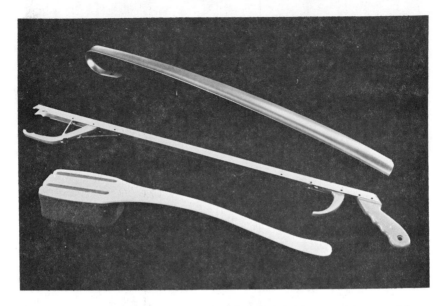

Figure 7-39. Long-handled sponge, long-handled holder or pickup, and long-handled shoehorn. Courtesy of J.A. Preston, New York.

midline of the body. The affected leg is crossed over the unaffected leg.

2. Pull the tongue of the shoe between the laces so that it will not be folded in the shoe.

3. Hold the short leg brace by the top portion of the inside metal bar. Swing the brace back and then forward so the heel is between the metal bars. Still holding onto the bar of the brace, turn the shoe inward so the toes will go in at a slight angle.

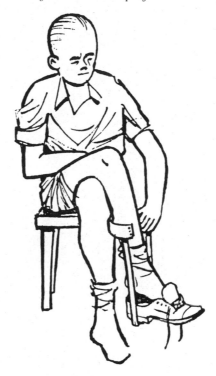

4. Pull the brace onto the leg as far as possible. Hold the brace in position by squeezing the crossbar between the legs and insert a long-handled shoehorn under the heel.

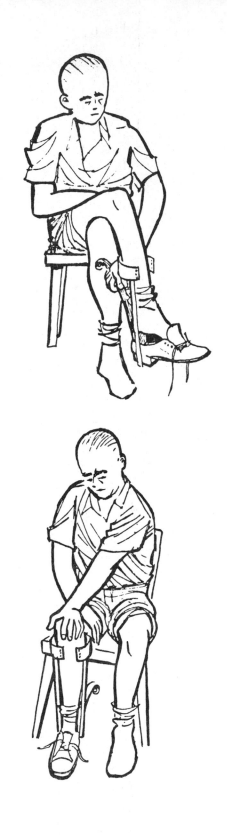

5. While holding the inside metal bar, uncross the affected leg and place the foot on the floor. Alternately, press down on the knee and move the shoehorn back and forth with the unaffected hand until the foot slips into the shoe. Talcum powder in the shoe will make it easier to slip on.

6. Fasten the laces and straps.

Procedure for Removing Shoes with Short Leg Brace

1. Cross the affected leg over the good leg.

2. Unfasten the straps and laces.

3. Push down on the brace until the shoe is off the foot.

Procedure for Fastening Shoelaces

A hemiplegic patient can learn to tie shoelaces in the regular manner; however, the following alternative, a one-looped bow with one lace, may be easier to learn and equally satisfactory.

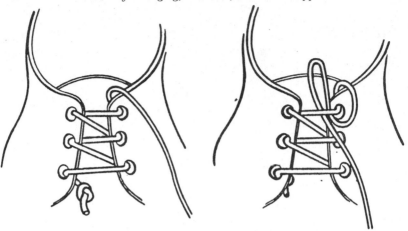

1. Lace shoes by putting a knot in one end of the lace. Lace the other end through each hole, beginning at the hole nearest the toe of the shoe. Proceed to top, always lacing from top to the tongue.

2. When shoe is laced to top, form a small loop with free end. To form a knot, place loop over and under top lace near the last threaded eye. Draw loop tight to the shoe.

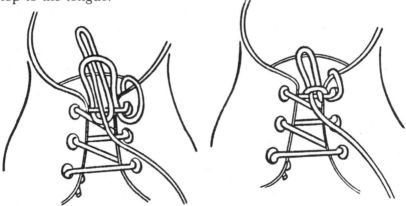

3. With remaining free end, make another loop and draw through first loop.

4. Draw this loop tightly to the shoe to fasten.

5. This bow can be unfastened by pulling on the end of the lace. This makes a very firm fastening.

Alternatives to Shoelaces

1. Hooks and a permanent knot. A permanent knot may be used with shoe hooks. The knot is slipped over the hook to close and may be removed for opening.

2. Elastic shoelaces, zipper locks, and Velcro fastenings may be purchased at a local shoe store and used with any laced shoe. It is also possible to purchase shoes with zipper, Velcro, or snap fastenings rather than the traditional laces. Any one of these methods eliminates the need for shoe tying.

General Considerations

Independent self-care is possible for many hemiplegics. Most hemiplegics can learn to do some of the daily living activities. The patient must learn to do with one arm and leg what he has previously done with two.

It is important for nurses, the patient's family, and workers to understand the reasons for training the patient to do his own daily living activities. Some suggestions were listed for teaching the hemiplegic patient. It may be necessary to adjust the methods for individual patients.

In teaching the patients one-handed activities, some general considerations are the following:

1. It is important that the instructor know the procedure thoroughly before attempting to teach patients.
2. It is important to know the patient's abilities and limitations in order to teach the patient effectively.
3. Verbal directions must be clear and concise, and the same directions should be given each time and repeated until the patient understands. Visual directions or demonstrations may be needed to clarify verbal instructions. Some patients become confused, so it is important for the nurse to be patient when instructing.
4. Most activities should be done with the patient seated rather than standing. In this way, he can concentrate on the immediate task and not be concerned about falling.
5. At first, articles to be used should be placed within easy reach of the patient. As he improves, he may become responsible for securing his own articles.

6. He should be encouraged and permitted to do as much for himself as possible. Each nurse or family member should expect the same degree of independence.
7. No adapted equipment should be furnished unless absolutely necessary.
8. Learning to perform self-care activities with one hand is sometimes fatiguing and frustrating. Beginning with one or two activities is important. As these skills are mastered and general strength increases, the patient should add new skills.
9. When teaching a patient self-care activities, the staff members should provide the opportunity to perform these tasks regularly each day.
10. If there is a visual problem, it may be necessary to call attention to both sides of the body when performing an activity.

The program of rehabilitation for a hemiplegia must be concerned mainly with the uninvolved side with the goals of ambulation and self-care. To prepare for ambulation, exercise for the uninvolved side must be vigorous, progressive, unassisted, short, and frequently repeated. This is best achieved by a program of standing exercises. As the patient begins to walk, he should retain his specific hemiplegia gait pattern and not attempt to simulate a normal gait. The patient must be trained in self-care activities with the use of the uninvolved arm. The hemiplegic patient should be protected against secondary disabilities.

ORGANIC MENTAL IMPAIRMENT

It is most important to remember that a disease that is primarily a motor disability can cause a mental impairment as a secondary result. In many elderly people there is an organic mental impairment, commonly called senility. It is very difficult to separate the motor disability from mental impairment, but the staff must be cognizant of its importance in the rehabilitation of the elderly patient.

Definition

A simple definition of the term organic mental impairment is any impairment of mental function caused by organic disorders of the brain. For a better understanding of mental impairment, they have been classified into types:

1. Disturbances of consciousness — people go to sleep or go into a coma or stupor, which could be for a very short period of time, minutes or hours, or days.
2. Lack of communication ability.
3. Disturbance of memory and thinking.

These symptoms are usually seen in patients who are mentally retarded or senile and who have organic mental syndromes. They are recognized by the following characteristics:

1. Disorientation as to time and space
2. Impairment of memory
3. Diminished length of memory span

The preceding symptoms are frequently seen in patients who have had strokes, and if this is the case, some improvements may be made during rehabilitation. If no improvement is shown quickly, then it is safe to say that it is an organic mental syndrome. In this case, there is little that can be done. Understanding is the one thing that can help staff members do a better job.

Emotional Disturbances

1. Apathetic or depressed patient — in this emotional disturbance, patients are just not interested in anything; they must be pushed to do their daily activities and exercises.
2. Irritable patient — these patients are problems because they are always against anything suggested. They are irritated by everything they do and everything the staff does to try to rehabilitate them.
3. Anxious patient — these patients have a poor attention span but are always very eager to perform exercises and activities; however, they frequently tend to do things too fast. They fall behind in their achievements, activities of daily living, and locomotion.

It is evident that the rehabilitation worker must be able to recognize the patients with different mental or neurological disorders. As a result, the management of the patient consists of two phases:

1. The patients/residents must be given an adequate amount of stimulation.
2. They must not be subject to excessive demands.

It has been discovered that the elderly patient with signs of organic brain disturbances or impairments, if left in bed with no attention given to them, gradually becomes incontinent, more withdrawn, more disoriented, and more confused. However, if this patient is included in a daily routine that brings him in contact with other people and requires some activity on his part, it will result in his attention span improving. His memory and orientation improves, and in many cases, he functions so well that he does not need the attention that was formerly required.

A word of caution must be given at this time. If the activity is too much, and if this patient meets too many people, then he will become completely disoriented and need far more help than before. Everything must be done gradually, and the patient must be carefully watched.

Brain Damaged Patients

Most brain damaged patients have a decrease in their ability to assimilate information and experiences in order to learn. Rehabilitation goals emphasize learning. In these patients, one must study carefully the intellectual deficit and the lack of ability to process information. In order to understand a patient, the staff member learn symptoms or signs that indicate the amount and source of brain damage.

Areas of Intellectual Functioning

1. Symbolic — This involves use of language, numbers, concepts, and ideas. Any performance in this area requires ability to receive, comprehend, and respond in language and numerical figures. Symbolic functioning is impaired if there is damage to the dominant left cerebral hemisphere, if the person is right-handed.
2. Perceptual — This involves the discrimination and appreciation of form, distance, position, and movements. These functions occur through the right cerebral hemisphere. An example is the

right-handed left hemiplegic who finds it difficult to steer his wheelchair well enough to avoid hitting the door frame.

Signs or symptoms of brain damage are as follows:

1. Have problems receiving and transmitting communications.
2. Tend to show difficulties in making judgments.
3. Problems in activities requiring drawing and geometric forms, and in maintaining upright position while ambulating.
4. Difficulty in positioning the involved arm.
5. Putting on a shirt correctly is difficult.

It has been shown that those working with the brain damaged patients need to guide the form of their communications by those defects.

One of the problems that is not clearly understood but does exist is that brain damaged patients cannot learn well because of their memory losses, that is, losses in the ability to retain a response from one occasion to another. One technique that has proven successful for this type of patient is to put everything down on cards with symbols and letters. Especially in the field of self-care.

To help the worker and to clarify the information, the following chart might be helpful:

Rehabilitation Management for Patients with Brain Damage

1. Symbolic (left brain, right hemiplegia)
   a. Simplify and reduce symbol clues and directions.
   b. Use short symbols and standard terms.
2. Perceptual (right brain, left hemiplegia)
   a. Evaluate carefully.
   b. Emphasize symbols, clues, and directions.
      Note: This is for the right-handed. The reverse is true for left-handed people.
3. Memory
   a. Check auditory attention span.
   b. Check separately pre- and post-learning and recall.
   c. Maximize external clues.

It is helpful to the person working with the patient if a psychologist is available to make some tests and share the results with the worker.

Some tests available for use in three areas are the following:

1. Intelligence

2. Personality
3. Special for the brain damaged patient

The patient with brain damage has an especially hard time reaching the maximum of return. The staff's ability to understand them is the most important requirement in achieving the maximum from rehabilitation.

MUSCULOSKELETAL IMPAIRMENT

For a person to function to the fullest in rehabilitation, understanding of the disease is very important. Mental disorders have already been discussed. Now we move to skeletal and muscular disorders.

Arthritis

Arthritis is inflammation of one or more joints. If the condition persists for a long period of time, it is called chronic arthritis, of which there are three types: (1) rheumatoid arthritis; (2) osteoarthritis and (3) gouty arthritis.

RHEUMATOID ARTHRITIS. To manage and treat this type of patient better, and explanation of what is happening to the joints as a result of the disease is advisable. There are basically five stages.

FIRST STAGE. Inflammation of the synovial membrane with or without excessive secretion of synovial fluid into the joint space.

SECOND STAGE. The synovial membrane proliferates and thickens. This causes swelling of the joint, which is usually accompanied by pain.

THIRD STAGE. The synovial membrane grows into the joint space, covers the surfaces of the cartilage, and destroys it by pressure.

FOURTH STAGE. The bony surfaces of the adjacent bones are now exposed, and the joint space is diminshed as a result of the lost articular cartilage.

FIFTH STAGE.
1. If there is no secretion of synovial fluid because of complete destruction of synovial membrane, the exposed bony surfaces will grow together. This is called ankylosis.
2. If there is sufficient secretion of synovial fluid to lubricate the

bony surfaces and prevent ankylosis, there may be subluxation of the joint depending upon the amount of looseness in the joint capsule and surrounding ligaments.

Use of the joint may cause additional damage, along with swelling and pain.

Pain is usually the cause of lack of use of the body part. The voluntary immobilization then leads to atrophy of surrounding muscles, osteoporosis of adjoining bones, and limitation of range of motion by contractures.

In rheumatoid arthritis, there may be a remission in any stage. Thus, it is apparent that a specific rehabilitation program must be made for each affected joint at each stage of development.

At this time, it is well known that limitation of joint range of motion and joint deformity are common features of rheumatoid arthritis. The most frequent disorders are flexion contractures of the hip, the knees, and the elbows. This means that the hips, knees, and the elbows cannot be fully extended. The arm cannot be raised due to the limitation of motion in the shoulder joint. Fingers cannot be fully flexed because there are contractures. Rehabilitation must aim toward restoration of the joint movements. The goal is full range of motion, but sometimes this cannot be attained, and staff members must do what they can to make the patient comfortable, as well as functional.

Osteoarthritis

Osteoarthritis is a disorder of mechanical origin. It is wear and tear, usually in weight-bearing joints, that occurs in late middle age. Elderly persons who have loose ligaments, joint capsules, and/or atrophied muscles are very vulnerable to minor injuries. Osteoarthritis frequently occurs as a result of trauma from heavy loads and overuse. Osteoarthritis is not primarily an infectious disease. It is different from rheumatoid arthritis in that the changes occur in cartilage. The synovial membrane is not affected. There is an erosion of cartilage and diminution of joint space and a loosening of ligaments and joint capsule, leading to a degree of joint instability. This leads to thickening of the margins of the capsule and spur formation of the bone. The irritative effect of the spurs and the irregular motions in an unstable joint lead to irritation of the surrounding soft tissue. The inflammation will subside upon rest. Pain is present upon initial movements but shortly subsides to a tolerable level.

Gouty Arthritis

Since gouty arthritis is a rarer disease and does not frequently come under rehabilitation, this will not be detailed closely. It is a disturbance of uric acid metabolism, causing small deposits of urates in the bone or soft tissue near the joint surface. These deposits may break through the cartilage and cause damage. Joint activity aggravates this condition. Its onset is sudden, usually in the first joint of the big toe. Diet and medication are usually effective.

REHABILITATION OF MUSCULOSKELETAL DISORDERS

In musculoskeletal disorders, there are two elements that must be considered: (1) pain and (2) muscular weakness.

PAIN. Pain is the most common and most disabling complaint of patients with chronic arthritis. Pain may be present in or near the affected joints, or it may be generalized and difficult to relate to a particular joint. Pain may be present while the patient is at rest. It may be produced and aggravated by voluntary as well as passive motion.

MUSCULAR WEAKNESS. Muscular weakness is common in rheumatoid arthritis. Atrophy and weakness are caused by disuse. If pain is present, the patients tend to not use their muscles, thus developing muscular weakness. If pain is eliminated then use of muscles will soon regain the musclar strength.

The challenges confronting the staff in rehabilitation are that rest will relieve pain and bring a reduction to the disease of the painful joint but that the many joints that are not affected by arthritis, when they are not in use, will lose muscular strength and mobility.

Another method to immobilize the affected joint is by use of bandages. If immobilization is carried out, regardless of method, it is essential that range of motion be done on the immobilized joints. One method that has been found successful has been to put the patients into hot tubs of water and exercise them at that time. This will help to prevent contractures and will be less painful than doing exercises in bed.

There are times, if the joint pain is due to mechanical causes, such as instability due to ligament destruction or erosion of cartilage, that immobilization can be carried out without undue pain. For example, if it is in the wrist, you can use a wrist strap or splint. If it is in the knee, knee braces can be used. The same applies to the ankle, with the use of an ankle support. This will be taken up more fully in the section on physical therapy.

Locomotion for the Arthritic

The emphasis is on the arthritis patient. The patient with arthritis can remain independent longer through early rehabilitation. Losing the ability to ambulate is perhaps the most discouraging aspect of this disease. The arthritis patient who resigns himself to a life in a wheelchair and progressive discomforts is admitting defeat. This prevents adjustment to the disease. Prevention should be emphasized, not resignation.

One of the most important ways to help arthritic patients is the use of protective devices. For example, consider a patient who is unstable due to deformed knees and ankles but whose hips and spine are not involved. If the knees and ankles are stabilized in functional position, the patient can then use the normal areas to learn how to transfer from bed to standing position or from chair to standing. Listed are a few devices used in rehabilitation procedure.

1. Special shoes for weight bearing
2. Use of leather anklets
3. Use of exercises to overcome contractures
4. Long or short leg braces for support

With the use of these supportive measures, patients can be taught to ambulate although their gaits may be awkward because they swing their lower extremities from the hips. It might also be necessary to use crutches for safe ambulation.

The patients with lower extremity difficulties that use the protective devices must be taught how to get out of bed fully braced. The patient is taught to roll over on his stomach and slide his feet off the bed. As his feet touch the floor, he stabilizes himself on his elbows and then stands erect by extending his hips.

Self-Care

Self-care for the arthritic patient who has serious problems of the upper extremities involves use of many new devices developed in rehabilitation. Following is a small list of the more common devices. Others are constantly being developed for people with special needs.

1. A sponge rubber handle for eating utensils.
2. Long-handled utensils (comb, toothbrush, shoehorn).
3. Stocking holders with garter clamps to pull up stockings.
4. Laces of shoes.
5. Zippers instead of buttons or laces.

The occurrence of pain in arthritis is so common that its importance must be mentioned here again. Since no one else can feel the patient's pain, many people working with the arthritic patient push him to do things that are very harmful and totally unsafe. The arthritic patient must make many adjustments to his handicaps.

REFERENCES

1. Psychologic Aspects, by Martha Storandt. In *The Care of the Geriatric Patient,* edited by Franz U. Steinberg. C.V. Mosby Co., St. Louis, 1976.
2. Neurologic Aspects, by William B. Hardin. In *The Care of the Geriatric Patient,* edited by Franz U. Steinberg. C.V. Mosby Co., St. Louis, 1976.
3. *Aging and Mental Health,* by Robert N. Butler and Myrna I. Lewis. C.V. Mosby Co., St. Louis, 1977.
4. *Rehabilitation, A Manual for the Care of the Disabled and Elderly,* by Gerald G. Hirshberg, Leon Lewis, and Dorothy Thomas. J.B. Lippincott Co., 1964.
5. *Restorative Medicine in Geriatrics,* by Michael M. Dasco. Charles C Thomas, Springfield, Illinois, 1963.
6. Long-Term Health Care, by John K. Iglehard, The Problem that Won't Go Away, *National Journal,* November 1977, pp. 1725-27.
7. J.A. Prestion Corp., Fifth Avenue, New York, illustrations of rehabilitative equipment.
8. Everest and Jennings Co., Los Angeles, details on wheelchairs.
9. Material from a seminar given by Division of Health, Department of Health and Social Services, Madison, Wisconsin, on Self-Care Activities for the Hemiplegic Patient, University of Wisconsin.

Chapter 8

SPECIFIC AREAS OF REHABILITATION

INTRODUCTION

THIS chapter will explore the many areas of rehabilitation. Each specialty will be detailed. All members of the rehabilitative team are specialists in their own field. They know what to do. The purpose of this chapter is to give a nurse or aide or any staff worker an introduction to each of the fields that compose the rehabilitation team. We have discussed the purpose of rehabilitation: all specialists work on the restoration of a patient until they (the patients) have reached the maximum that can be achieved.

PHYSICAL THERAPY

Physical therapy is the treatment of disease, disability, and injury to relieve pain, develop or restore function, and maintain maximum performance using the physical energies of massage, heat, water, radiant energy (exclusive of x-ray and radium), electricity, and ultrasound and the physiological energy of exercise. The physical therapist makes diagnostic and prognostic muscle, nerve, joint, and functional ability tests; makes use of equipment such as ultraviolet machines; directs and aids patients in active and passive exercises, muscle re-education, self-care activities, transfers, gait, and functional training by utilizing pulleys, weights, steps, and inclined surfaces; gives whirlpool baths and applies hot and cold packs; directs patients in care and uses of wheelchairs, braces, canes, crutches and prosthetic and orthotic devices; gives instructions in posture and procedures to be continued at home; and keeps records of treatments given and patients' responses and progress.

Physical therapy makes use of naturally occurring phenomena, which is one of the oldest methods in the field of medicine. The warming rays of the sun, the flow of water, and the use of electricity are examples. These forces help in circulation, change general body metabolism, relieve nerve irritation, or stimulate nerve function, inhibit growth of germs, sometimes destroy them, and, as a result,

239

speed up repair of injured tissues, restore function, relieve pain, and improve the entire body.

Physical therapy is not a new field. It is an old profession using physical agents in conjunction with medical and surgical measures after a diagnosis has been made. One of the most important aspects of physical therapy is the physical and physiological effects that can be produced by physical agents. Any form of physical energy applied to the body exerts first a physical action known as the "primary physical effects," which, in turn, brings on the "secondary physiological effects." Thus, the influence on organic or functional changes in the body will be in direct proportion to the extent of the primary physical changes.

The following table gives some idea of the physical agents used and their primary and secondary physical and physiological effects.

PHYSICAL AGENT	PRIMARY PHYSICAL EFFECT	SECONDARY PHYSIOLOGICAL EFFECTS
Hot water baths Hot packs Infrared lamps	Thermal	Hyperemia Relief of pain Relaxation of muscles
Diathermy		Attenuation of growth of germs
Ethyl chloride spray Cold packs Direct application of ice	Reduction of temperature	Diminished formation of tissue fluid. Constriction of vessels Relief of pain Relaxation of muscles
Ultrasound	Thermal Mechanical	Hyeremia Mobilization of tissue fluids Relief of pain Relaxation of muscles
Sun	Photochemical	Hyperemia

Carbon arc lamps		Increased red and
Mercury vapor arc		white blood cells
		Activation of
		vitamin D
Direct electrical current	Electrochemical	Diminished pain
rent		Ion transfer
Low frequency current	Electrokinetic	Contraction of innervated and
rent		nervated and
		denervated muscles
Massage	Kinetic	Increase of venous
		and lymphatic
		flow
		Prevents contractures
		tures
		Stimulation of
		superficial reflexes

Thus, basic changes and improvements can be achieved by hot and cold applications, active and passive exercises, and massage, plus a kind and understanding person. The philosophy of a physical therapist in treating a patient is, "Do as much as he can, as well as he can, for improvement, as fast as he can."

Since rehabilitation means the restoration of an ill or injured patient to self-sufficiency, in the shortest possible time this covers all concepts from the restoration of specific function to actual recovery of capacity for earning a living in the community outside the nursing home. Too often, many people think that rehabilitation and physical therapy are the same when, in fact, physical therapy is only one field or tool in rehabilitating a patient. There are many essential tools required to implement the rehabilitative process. These will be discussed in this chapter.

It is necessary to have a team approach in the field of rehabilitation in order to have the most successful program. Physical therapists have a unique contribution to make to rehabilitation. They have a background in kinesiology; they have knowledge of motion, which involves an understanding of the nervous system the biomechanics of joints, and the musculoskeletal system as a whole. If there is a patheological or traumatic condition, the physical therapist is qualified by special education to restore motion and muscular strength, which are the most important elements in rehabilitation and self-care, in getting patients up and doing things for themselves. With his knowledge of anatomy, physiology, and pathology, the physical therapist who realizes the emotional impact of a disability is in a position to exert a strong force in the rehabilitation of patients/residents in a nursing home.

In rehabilitation it has been repeatedly pointed out that a proper evaluation must be made prior to any definite rehabilitation services being started. The physical therapist can act as the evaluator because of his basic education and professional knowledge.

In a nursing home that has a physical therapist on its staff, the following procedure is carried out: When a new patient checks into the nursing home, his physical condition is evaluated by the physical therapist. This evaluation report is then discussed with the patient's physician. If physical therapy is prescribed, the program is carried out in the overall treatment plan. If no physical therapy treatment is prescribed, but in the evaluation it was indicated that the patient could benefit from the nursing home rehabilitation program, which encourages self-care and physical independence, then it should be initiated.

The next step is to have a consultation with the director of nursing services. Physical therapy carries out their phase of rehabilitation and nursing service carries out their part.

In-service training programs are arranged to give the nursing staff adequate instructions on their phase of rehabilitation. Periodically, the patient receives new evaluations, and changes are made accordingly. Thus, every patient in the home gets the benefits of rehabilitation. Progress notes are made on patients' charts to indicate the goals of the program and progress made. The physician in charge checks the program and makes suggestions that he feels will benefit the patient. Communication is made whenever necessary between the physical therapist and director of rehabilitative nursing. This is one example of a two member team in rehabilitation.

What can be done if the nursing home does not have a staff physical therapist? A physical therapist can be called in as a consultant, or could come in once a week to do the evaluations, set up the program, and give in-service training to the staff in the three basic fundamental procedures that are easily available, which are the following:

PHYSICAL AGENT	MODALITY	EFFECT
1. Cold	Ice Any cold substance	Relief of pain Decrease in spasticity Relaxes muscles Prevents edema
2. Heat	Hot packs Infrared lamps Hot bath	Increased circulation Connective tissue is easier to stretch Relief of pain Muscle relaxation

3. Exercise	Active and passive
	  range of motion
	
	Stretching
	Relaxation
	
	Special
		Improved vascular
		  tone
		Improved respiration
		Improved posture
		Improved mobility
		Increased strength
		Improved coordina-
		  tion
		Improved endurance
		Muscle imbalance
		  corrected
		Improvment of —
		  transfer activities
		  gait and ambula-
		  tion
		  functional ac-
		  tivities
		  activities of daily
		  living

Physical therapists can function as educators as well as consultants. They can and should teach in two areas:

1. They can teach basic procedures —
    a. Body mechanics
    b. Transfer techniques
    c. General walking activities
    d. Positioning of patients for specific diseases or disabilities
    e. Activities of daily living

This is for all members of the nursing staff, and all should be required to learn this material. As a result, all personnel of the nursing home who work with patients will have acquired sufficient basic knowledge that leads to an improved job for the patient and for the staff worker.

2. The physical therapist can teach members of the nursing staff the procedures to employ with a specific patient on a continuing basis during the intervals between the physical therapist's visits. In this manner, the efficiency of his direct service is multiplied.

As has been pointed out earlier, the goal of rehabilitation in the nursing home environment presents a challenge with which only a rehabiliation team can cope. No such team can be effective if it does not include a physical therapist because his special knowledge in kinesiology, anatomy, and exercises qualifies him to bring to the team a unique understanding of motion that is vital in the fight for physical independence.

Posture and Body Mechanics

The personnel of a nursing home should recognize the need for integrating body mechanics and posture in all activities. The posture of different parts of the body have a relationship to the way in which the skeletal, muscular, nervous, and other body systems function. The way a person stoops, reaches, lifts, carries, sits, and stands may increase or decrease fatigue. By understanding the normal use of the body and applying this knowledge to his own posture, an individual will be more effective in all of his work, be he patient or worker.

To Help Develop Good Body Mechanics

1. Keep chest up and forward
2. Maintain normal spinal curves.
3. Stand with feet separated, toes pointing ahead.
4. Keep weight balanced over base of support.
5. When possible, use leg and thigh muscles instead of back lifting.

Seven Basic Steps to Lifting

1. Get as close as possible to the object to be lifted.
2. Divide the weight between both hands.
3. Lift by flexing elbows and bringing weight against the body.

4. Flex hips and knees if weight is lower than hand reach, keeping back as straight as possible (crouch position).
5. Stabilize trunk by setting abdominal muscles and back extensors.
6. Flex elbows, bring weight up against the body, straighten hips and knees by use of the large extensor muscles.
7. Keep work at elbow height when possible. Never twist torso; pivot on heels, if necessary, to have feet pointed in direction of motion.

Body Alignment and Positioning of Patients

Patients must be positioned in a comfortable position to prevent contractures and deformities. Some will need specific positions, such as amputee, stroke patients, arthritic cases, etc. The following gives a better understanding in this.

1. Equipment that can be used
   a. Pillows
   b. Footboards
   c. Knotted ropes
   d. Sandbags
   e. Trochanter or hip bone, use towels, and hand rolls
   f. Overhead trapeze
2. Terminology
   a. Supine — lying on back
   b. Sidelying — lying on one side
   c. Prone — lying face down
3. Supine
   a. Maintain normal alignment of head and the cervical, thoracic, and lumbar physiology curves.
      (1) Use a small pillow under the head.
      (2) Use a small pad under the lumbar spine.
   b. Feet at right angles.
      (1) Use footboard and towel roll to prevent lateral rotation.
      (2) Place covers over the footboard to eliminate pressure on toes.
      Note: Adjustable footboard keeps patients feet aligned in

upper postion (Fig. 8-1).

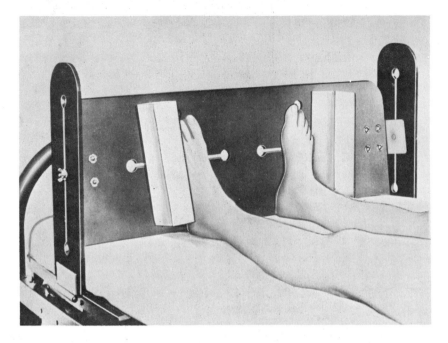

Figure 8-1. Adjustable footboard with antirotation supports. Courtesy of J.A. Preston, New York.

    c. Knees in slight flexion unless contraindicated.
       (1) Use towel roll for this purpose.
    d. Prevent lateral rotation of lower extremities.
    e. Prop the arms part of the time in abduction, alternating external and internal rotation by supporting forearms with pillows forward, then backward (can place hand on chest for forward rotation).
    f. Towel roll on chest to support wrists and fingers in functional position. (This is a must for arthritic patients.)
4. Sidelying
    a. Small pillow under the head and neck to align them with spine for stability.
    b. Pillow between legs, which may be flexed at hips and knees, if not contraindicated.
    c. Pillow tucked under back for stability.
    d. Two pillows in front of chest to support uppermost arm,

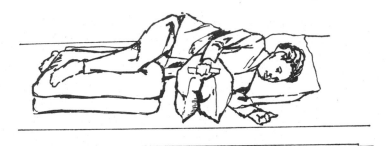

Figure 8-2. Full side lying. Towel rolls or sandbags commonly used in supporting body segments against gravity. Note roll in hand for fingers. Towels used to support upper leg and arm in side lying.

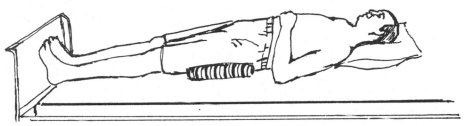

Figure 8-3. Use of trochanter roll on side of hip and footboard prevents external rotation, plantar flexion, and foot drop.

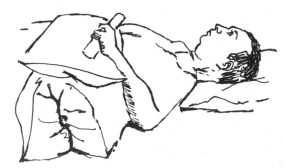

Figure 8-4. Supine position. Pillows or towels placed to reduce shoulder internal rotation and adduction tightness and/or to prevent additional tightness. Roll in hand prevents finger tightness.

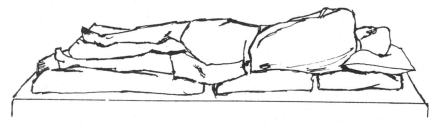

Figure 8-5. Proper side-lying position.

if desired.

5. Positioning for Special Conditions
  a. Hemiplegia
    (1) Arm abducted with changes in rotation when supine.
    (2) Prevent pronation of forearm by use of towel roll between body and supinated forearm.
    (3) Prevent flexion of wrist, fingers, and thumb by use of towel roll on chest when supine, on supporting pillows when sidelying.
    (4) No towel roll under involved knee.
    (5) Prevent flexion, abduction, and lateral rotation of leg and thigh by constant use on trochanter with towel rolls when supine.
    (6) Prevent foot drop. Use of footboard, or bivalved plaster cast.
  b. Paraplegia
    (1) Prevent hip flexion contracture. Keep hips and knees extended.
    (2) Prevent equinus deformity. Footboard and bivalved casts.
  c. Arthritic Cases
    (1) Prevent acquisition of an unbalanced hand.
        Towel roll on chest, cock-up splint.
    (2) Prevent flexion contractures of hips and knees.
        Keep them straight.
  d. Amputees
    (1) Prevent flexion and abduction contractures of hip joint in above knee (A.K.) amputations. Do not permit, at any time, propping of stump up on pillow.
    (2) Prevent knee flexion contracture if below knee (B.K.). Keep knee straight.

Bed Patient

In addition to general positioning, there are special problems and precautions needed for the care of a bed patient.

1. Pay attention to the position of joints to prevent strain and possible subluxation and to the position of the extremities to prevent contractures.

2. Change the position of the patient regularly, every two to four

hours — every two hours if the patient is helpless and every four hours if he is able to shift his position slightly to relieve pressure on prominent bony areas such as sacrum, lateral hip, heels, and elbows (Figs. 8-6 and 8-7).

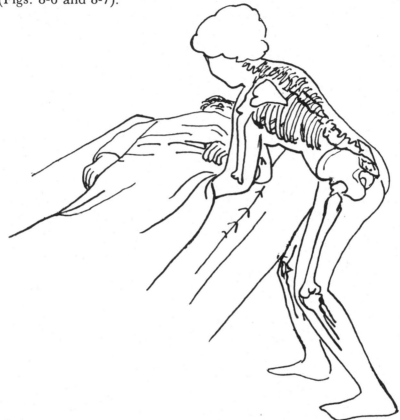

Figure 8-6. Moving bed patient to the side. Place one arm under head and shoulders. Place other arm under patient's waist. Flex hips and knees. Place one knee forward against bed. Keep shoulders taut. Shift weight from forward leg to back leg. Move hips and legs in line with upper trunk.

Helping a Patient into a Wheelchair

1. Place wheelchair at a 45-degree angle to bed on patient's strong side, facing foot of bed. Keep front corner of the chair as close to the bed as possible, with brakes locked and foot-rests up.
2. Have the patient sit up and swing his legs over the side of the bed. If he cannot do this himself, lock arms with him and bring

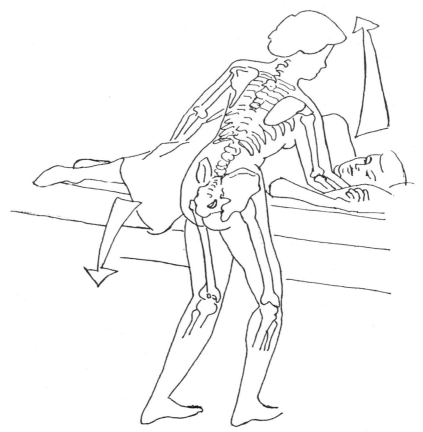

Figure 8-7. Moving patient from supine to sitting. Face patient. Support under neck and shoulders. Hold patient in bend of knees. Place forward leg against bed. Set trunk muscles. Shift weight from forward leg to back leg. Shift patient to sitting.

    him to a sitting position. With one of the assistant's arms under his knees, swing his legs over the side of the bed. Let the patient rest in this position.

3. Help the patient step to the floor. Place arms under both of his armpits with hands well onto his back. Keep his weight forward. Turn him so that the back of his legs are close to the chair. Have patient place hands on the arm of chair; move with him as he eases well back into the chair.

4. Adjust leg rests to support his legs and feet.

5. If the patient has a paralyzed arm, support it with a pillow or

sling.

6. Always be very careful when helping a patient into a wheelchair. An armchair can be used by the bed instead of a wheelchair. It should be heavy enough so that it will not slide and should have a firm seat. The height is very important to the patient.

Turning the Patient Away from Helper

1. Assist the patient to flex his knees.
2. Slip one arm under the back and far shoulder; place the other as far as possible under the thighs.
3. Lift and draw the far side of the patient closer so that he is gradually facing away.

Turning a Helpless Patient

1. Take two pillows to side of bed and place them near the helper.
2. Slip hand under patient's shoulders and hips and have the helper do the same on the other side.
3. On signal, move the patient to the helper's side of the bed.
4. Draw the patient's legs to the far side of the bed.
5. Place hands over the patients trunk well back of the far shoulder and hip; draw them closer while the helper pushes the knees.
6. Have your helper place pillows behind patient's back for stabilization.
7. Adjust the patient's head, shoulders, and arms.

Lifting a Patient Up in Bed

1. Remove all pillows but one from under patient's head.
2. Move remaining pillow up toward the head of the bed.
3. Assist patient to flex his knees and tell him to press his feet down on the bed.
4. Put one arm under patient's shoulders and the other under his thighs.
5. Have the helper do the same from the oppostie side and on signal partially lift and slide the patient toward the head of the bed. The

patient, if able, may place one arm under and around both helpers' shoulders.

Range of Motion

Range is the extent of movement within a given joint. *Motion* in a joint is achieved through the action of a muscle or a group of muscles. Each joint has a normal range, which can be measured by a goniometer.

DEFINITIONS OF JOINT MOVEMENTS

FLEXION. Bending.
EXTENSION. Straightening.
ABDUCTION. Moving the part away from the midline of the body.
ADDUCTION. Moving the part toward the midline of the body.
INTERNAL ROTATION. Limb or body part turns inward around its axis.
EXTERNAL ROTATION. Limb or body part turns outward around its axis.
CIRCUMDUCTION. Circular movement combining first four movements.

RANGE OF MOTION EXAMPLES

Head

FLEXION. Looking down, put chin on chest.
EXTENSION. Looking up at sky or ceiling.
ABDUCTION. To right, move ear toward right shoulder. To left, move ear toward left shoulder.

Shoulder

ELEVATION. Raise shoulder up, like in a shrug.
DEPRESSION. Push shoulder downward.
PROTRACTION. Move shoulder forward.
RETRACTION. Move shoulder backward.

Arm

FLEXION. Move arm forward and upward.
EXTENSION. Move arm downward and backward.
ABDUCTION. Move arm from body to shoulder height.
ADDUCTION. Move arm toward body across chest.
INTERNAL ROTATION. With arm at shoulder height and elbow flexed,

move forearm forward and downward.

EXTERNAL ROTATION. From internally rotated position, bring forearm upward and backward.

Forearm

FLEXION. Move palm of hand toward shoulder.

EXTENSION. Straighten elbow.

SUPINATION. With elbow flexed to 90 degrees, turn palm of hand up.

PRONATION. From supinated position, turn palm downward.

Wrist

FLEXION. Move palm of hand toward forearm.

EXTENSION. Move back of hand toward forearm.

RADIAL DEVIATION. Move thumb side of hand toward side of forearm.

ULNAR DEVIATION. Move little finger side of hand toward side of forearm.

Fingers and Thumb

FLEXION. Make a fist, bring thumb over clinched fingers.

EXTENSION. Straighten fingers and thumb, keeping latter next to hand.

ABDUCTION. Separate fingers and thumb from the extended position.

ADDUCTION. Bring fingers and thumb together in extended position.

OPPOSITION. Touch thumb tip to little finger tip.

Hip

FLEXION. Raise thigh forward and upward until parallel with floor, knee flexed.

EXTENSION. Move lower extremity downward and backward.

ABDUCTION. Move extremity away from body, keeping trunk erect.

ADDUCTION. Move extremity toward midline of body and across it.

INTERNAL ROTATION. With knee flexed, turn knee toward midline.

EXTERNAL ROTATION. With knee flexed, turn knee away from midline.

Knee

FLEXION (PRONE POSITION). Lift leg upward, keep thigh on surface.

EXTENSION (SITTING POSITION). Straighten knee.

Ankle

FLEXION (DORISFLEXION). Move top of foot toward leg.
EXTENSION (PLANTAR FLEXION). Move top of foot away from leg.
EVERSION. Turn sole of foot away from midline.
INVERSION. Turn sole of foot toward midline.

Toes

FLEXION. Curl toes downward.
EXTENSION. Pull toes upward.

Trunk

FLEXION. Supine, hips and knees flexed, feet flat on surface, stretch arms forward and try to come to a sitting position, hold to the count of five.
EXTENSION. Prone, chin tucked, head pushed backward, arms at sides, shoulders retracted, lift trunk not more than 3 to 4 inches, hold to the count of five.

Exercise

1. Definitions
   a. Exercise — to set in motion.
   b. Therapeutic or remedial or corrective exercise — the scientific application of bodily movements designed specifically to maintain or to restore normal function to diseased or injured muscles, nerves, and joints and to prevent deformities.
2. Types of contractions
   a. Isotonic (polymetric) — tone remains the same, but length changes.
      (1) Concentric (shortening) — the muscle shortens in spite of the resistance or load. Force exerted is greater than resistance, e.g. quadriceps when ascending steps.
      (2) Eccentric (lengthening) — the contracting muscle lengthens, the load is greater than the force, e.g. quadriceps when descending stairs.
   b. Isometric (monometric) — length remains the same, but tone is increased.
      (1) Little or no joint movement is present, e.g. contraction of

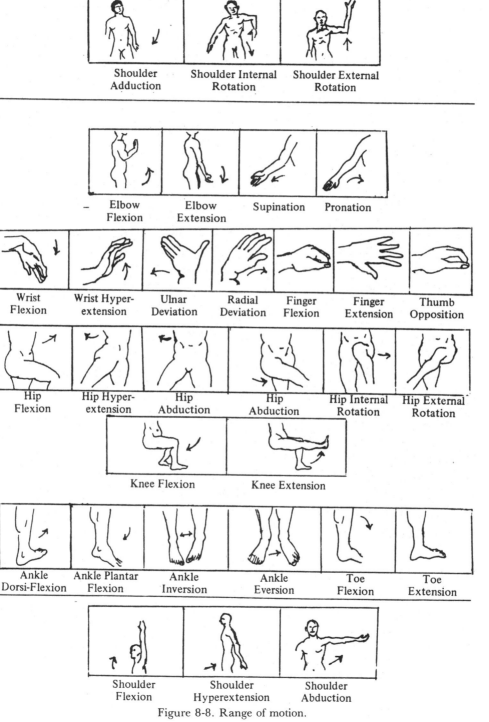

Figure 8-8. Range of motion.

muscles when an extremity is encased in a plaster cast or movement of joint is prevented manually or by a mechanical device.

(2) Also called static contraction or muscle setting.

(3) Reciprocal movement is the immediate reverse action, e.g. walking pattern, flexion and extension of elbow.

3. Classification of exercises
    a. Passive exercises — patient is completely relaxed; movement through R.O.M. is done by the physical therapist or one who has been instructed in how to do these exercises.
    b. Stretching (forced passive exercises) — patient is relaxed, restricted R.O.M. is forced by operator to stretch shortened structures, which may be muscles, tendons, ligaments, or joint capsules.
    c. Active exercises — patient voluntarily contracts muscles.
        (1) Assistive — assisted by operator to complete R.O.M. if muscle is weak.
        (2) Free — done by the patient alone.
        (3) Resistive — done by the patient against resistance offered by the operator or mechanical device such as weights.

Note: These exercises are done in various positions. For example, the patient is usually supine or prone for passive, assistive active, and stretching exercises, as well as for free active exercises. The positions will vary for resistive exercises. In-service training programs are essential to demonstrate techniques and to supervise practice.

4. Purpose of exercise
    a. Strengthen muscle groups — high, resistance, low frequency.
    b. Increase endurance — low resistance, high frequency.
    c. Coordination — practice and repetition.
    d. Increase speed — repetition and shorter intervals.
    e. General improvement of metabolism, circulation, relaxation and muscular tone.

Qualities of Muscles

1. Contraction — each fiber contracts to its maximum; as load increases, additional fibers contract.

2. Elasticity — ability to resume resting length after contraction.
3. Coordination — performance of a smooth, coordinated movement through neuromuscular control.

Pathology of Muscle Function

1. Weakness and atrophy — loss of muscle fibers.
2. Loss of elasticity — limitation of joint R.O.M., and inability to relax, which is neurological in origin.
   a. Spasm — a protective flex, usually the result of pain.
   b. Spasticity — result of a central nervous system lesion.
3. Loss of coordination — result of a cerebellar or basal ganglia lesion.
4. Contracture — diminished length of muscle fibers following long periods of immobilization, e.g. plaster casts. traction, or poor positioning.

Therapeutic Exercise to Improve Muscle Function

1. Weakness and atrophy — active and resistive exercises, concentric, isometric, and excentric.
2. Loss of elasticity
   a. Active relaxation of spasticity.
   b. Relief of pain for spasm.
   c. Stretching for contractures.
3. Loss of coordination — repetitious practice of a specific movement leads to precision of performance.

Physiology of Exercise

Exercises are essential to life and health. Circulation to the muscle tissue is improved by contraction and relaxation. Contraction squeezes the blood out; relaxation allows fresh blood to enter. Simultaneously, there is a pumping action to the veins and lymphatics. All processes such as breathing, blood flow, feeling of well-being, proper elimination, and good appetite are related. Muscles derive energy from stored carbohydrates and a lesser amount from fat and proteins. Proper diet is important.

Group Exercises

The purpose of a group exercise program for patients/residents of a nursing home is to get all of them involved in a daily active exercise program. This is for all ambulatory and nonambulatory patients. The program consists of active exercises done in the sitting position for wheelchair cases and others sitting in ordinary chairs. The exercises are primarily relaxation and conditioning types. Emphasis is on the large joints — shoulders, elbows, knees, and hips.

The program should be held daily, except on Saturday and Sunday, at about 11:30 AM, about one hour before lunchtime and should last about thirty minutes. The largest number of the nursing staff that is possible should be in attendance.

There is one important caution. Overexercise may result in a serious complication, e.g. the patient may have a heart condition. It is best to make sure that each patient has been evaluated by the physician as to their physical condition before participating in this program.

Method

All patients assemble in the dining room, or the activity room, or any large area sufficient to hold the class. Music is played for about five to ten minutes. This exercise period is made a part of the reality orientation program, which starts off by giving the day, month, and the year. Then, it is followed by current events, announcements of special interest, and then the exercises. After the program is over, the nurses pass out medications, since most of the resident/patients are in attendance.

Adapted Group Exercises for Nursing Home Program

Each exercise should be repeated ten times unless otherwise instructed. These are active exercises done by patients who are capable of complete or partial range of motion movements. They are designed to maintain or improve tolerance for activities and must be done routinely. The leader should avoid fatigue; each person has a different tolerance. Beginners should be advised to repeat each exercise only three times the first week, six the next, and ten the third.

Also, these beginners should meet with the leader after the exercise period to tell their reactions.

Adaptive Exercises

1. Abdominal breathing (diaphragmatic breathing). Inhale through the nose normally, letting the abdomen protrude. Exhale twice as long through mouth with lips pursed, pulling abdomen inward.
2. Shrug shoulders and tighten arm muscles (arms at sides with elbows straight); hold several seconds then let loose.
3. Drop chin on chest and curl trunk forward; breath out, do not bend at hips. Uncurl trunk, lift chin from chest, and breath in.
4. Fingertips on shoulders, arms shoulder high, make circles with elbows. Movement should be in shoulder joints only. Make five circles clockwise and five counterclockwise.
5. Start with arms at side. Move arm forward and upward until over the head, keeping elbows straight. Reach for the sky. Bring arms back to sides.
6. Feet flat on floor. Lift right foot off floor and straighten knee. Hold a few seconds, return foot to floor. Rest. Repeat with left foot and leg.
7. Feet flat on floor. Bring right knee up toward chest. Hold a few seconds. Return foot to floor. Rest. Repeat with left foot and leg.
8. Extend knees with heels resting on floor, pull feet up toward legs, then push feet down. Turn feet inward, then turn them outward, make circles with feet, five times clockwise and five times counterclockwise.

Results of Exercise Program

In nursing homes providing this exercise program, the staff has noticed a definite increase of patients doing more of their own activities of daily living. They have heard comments that the patients enjoyed the exercises. It has become a successful social occasion. The residents/patients have improved or maintained functions of activity, strength, mobility, and endurance.

It is important to remember the following:

1. The program must not be fatiguing; it must be simple; it must

be done daily; it must always be at the same time; it must keep the same format.

2. Before exercises are given, the instructor must —
   a. explain what he hopes to accomplish and how it will improve their pattern of living;
   b. explain normal reactions to exercise and also give signs of overexertion and fatigue;
   c. demonstrate each exercise; also, do them with the patient.
3. The instructor must be sure to —
   a. avoid pain as well as fatigue; he should tell patients to stop exercising if these occur and to report to him later;
   b. encourage all patients to participate; he should get their cooperation and help.

All members of the nursing staff must be trained to lead the program so that there is never a lack of a leader to guide it.

The nursing staff usually has the responsibility of carrying on rehabilitation of patients in a nursing home. In respect to goals of the program, the staff must think along the line of function. They should be satisfied with a range of motion that may be less than normal but that enables the limited joint to be functional for performing the activities of daily living.

To determine the extent of limited function a patient has before treatment and to check progress at intervals during the program, the following evaluation chart is given:

ACTIVITIES OF DAILY LIVING, AND EVALUATION
Check appropriate ( ) where requested.

Name_____Age_____Room_____

Method of Recording:　　　　　　　　　　　　　　Dates (Below)

    Yes — activity performed independently and safely.

    Poor — performed, but slowly and with difficulty.

    Not — cannot be performed.

    XX — not tested.

BED ACTIVITIES:

1. Move from side to side of bed. ( ) right; ( ) left
2. Roll from side to side. ( ) right; ( )left
3. Turn face down.
4. From lying to sitting position independently — using trapeze ( ) bed rails ( ) bed rope.

5. Sitting; move ( ) forward ( ) backward
6. Sitting; turn body and hang lower legs over side of the bed.
7. Reach articles on bedside table.
8. Operate signal light.

PERSONAL HYGIENE:

1. Comb or brush hair
2. Brush teeth
3. Remove and clean dentures
4. Shave or apply makeup
5. Clean or file fingernails
6. Wash face and hands
7. Bathe self: ( ) bed bath ( ) shower ( ) tub

DRESSING ACTIVITIES:

1. ( ) Put on ( ) take off — gown or pajamas
2. ( ) Put on ( ) take off — blouse or shirt
3. ( ) Put on ( ) take off — pants or skirt
4. ( ) Put on ( ) take off — dress
5. ( ) Put on ( ) take off — hose or socks
6. ( ) Put on ( ) take off — shoes
    ( ) Fasten shoes: ( ) lace and tie ( ) buckle
7. ( ) Put on ( ) take off — braces or appliances
8. Manage ( ) buttons ( ) snaps ( ) zippers ( ) hooks and eyes

EATING

1. Feed self
2. Handle eating tools
3. Pour water or milk from bottle
4. Drink from glass or cup
5. Spread butter on bread
6. Cut meat

HAND ACTIVITIES:

1. Write name and address
2. Open envelope and remove letter
3. Use telephone
4. Turn pages of book
5. Wind watch
6. Manage ( ) light switch ( ) doorknob ( ) house keys

WHEELCHAIR ACTIVITIES:

1. ( ) Move from bed to wheelchair and ( ) back
2. Propel wheelchair
3. Manage ( ) brakes ( ) locks
4. ( ) Open door ( ) go through door ( ) close door
5. ( ) Transfer from wheelchair to car ( ) back to wheelchair
6. Rise from wheelchair ( ) independently ( ) crutches or cane

STANDING, WALKING, STAIR CLIMBING:

1. Standing balance is adequate
2. Walking independently
   using ( ) crutches ( ) cane ( ) walker
3. Walk carrying a small package
4. ( ) Walk up normal height steps ( ) walk down steps
5. ( ) Walk up ramp ( ) walk down ramp.

Occupational Therapy

One way of understanding this area is to think of it as remedial activity. The activity is aimed at improving mental and physical disorders by active participation of the patient. Some of the basic aims of occupational therapy are as follows:

1. Restoration of function
2. Improvement and maintenance of physical function
3. Muscle compensation
4. Muscle strength development
5. Coordination
6. Dexterity
7. Correction of poor posture
8. Improved body mechanics
9. Enhanced work tolerance

The major goal of occupational therapy is to use arts and crafts to improve physical activity. This does not preclude the occupational therapist from using other physical and intellectual activities. One of the criticisms of the title occupational therapy is that it does not apply to occupations and the retraining of such but rather learning a new activities that have been lost and occupying the patient's time. The occupational therapist is a very diversified person, and in many nursing homes this person has taken over the recreational activities for which they are well qualified.

Rehabilitation by the occupational therapist starts when the patient has been admitted to the home and has been evaluated as to their needs. Thus, in many cases, they start giving activities to patients while they are bedfast. Treatment is prescribed individually for each patient.

The importance of activity is based on physical value and psychologic importance. Since each patient is different, some enjoy working in their rooms and others want to do their activity in a room where others are also working.

ARTS AND CRAFTS. Arts and crafts are the main media by which occupational therapists achieve their goals, aims, or objectives. The activity chosen for a patient is one that will improve one of their goals, for example, the strength of one of his upper extremities. Thus, carpentry may be selected because using a hammer or gardening using a hand tool strengthens the weakened extremity. By repetition, the patient will acquire coordination, dexterity, and strength.

Each activity must be analyzed for its physical and emotional values and its potential benefits to the patient. If the patient is sufficiently interested, then there will be benefits to the individual in (1) general strength, (2) balance, (3) attention span, (4) mental attitude, (5) physical dexterity, and (6) vision.

Frequently, physical therapy and occupational therapy will work together to try to use an activity that will benefit the patient in one specific area of malfunction.

Some activities in the field of arts and crafts are (1) weaving, (2) woodworking, (3) leather work, (4) ceramics, (5) needlecraft, and (6) general art.

The following example will serve to illustrate how an activity that a patient asks for may be beneficial after modification. A patient who has rheumatoid arthritis wants to knit but holds the knitting needles in a way that will further deform her hand. If she is taught to hold the knitting needles properly, the hand does not get further deformed, yet she gets satisfaction from knitting.

Weaving on a loom may be applied to nearly all disabilities. This activity can be graded in the strength required, and the loom can be adjusted according to the patient's needs along with weights or bars to add resistence. Weaving will increase range of motion for many arthritic patients. The use of lower level loom controls requires lifting the feet alternately, thus exercising the hip and knee extensors and the plantar flexors. Weaving has another dimension, as it helps a person to relieve themselves of hostility.

Most men do not care to use a loom; they prefer shop work. This field in many cases serves the same objectives as weaving. Woodwork can be graded in terms of strength required, the complexity for a specific patient, and its use for different parts of the anatomy. For example, wood may be cut on a bicycle saw, which requires reciprocal motion of the lower extremities and increases not only strength and range of motion but also body balance. Wood carving can improve hand strength, range of motion, and dexterity. A patient's grasp may be improved.

Leather lacing has proven successful with the hemiplegic patient. It can improve one-handed techniques, attention span, and general awareness and help the patient acquire visual field deficit compensation.

Writing is another difficult activity for many handicapped people. The use of an electric typewriter helps a person to write legibly and rapidly. Let the patient learn which is the best position for him to type.

MUSIC. Music is used by the entire nursing home to set the mood of the home, but music can accomplish many diversified results. It is both a physical and mental stimulus that has benefits for all people, including nursing home patients. The occupational therapist who is also the recreational director can provide opportunities for all patients to participate in musical activities. The therapist can record their music with a record player for replay in the activity room or could organize a live music group for singing and playing instruments. One nursing home formed a church choir, which started with only six voices and grew to twenty-two in a few weeks. They met every day for rehearsals and have become a social event in the nuring home.

Another nursing home nearby started a band. Two patients started the idea; one played the piano and the other the violin. They played for the activity programs, dinners, and any other time they were asked. Later, another woman joined them and brought her horn. Soon others joined them and they had eight players. The two nursing home groups got together, rented a bus, and started playing for groups all over the town.

GAMES. Games can be used for socialization, coordination, and increased attention span. Among the games most popular are card games of all kinds, chess, and checkers. Puzzles are also a popular activity and can be used for developmental purposes. If larger physical activities are desired, the therapist can try table tennis or shuffleboard. These have proven successful as part of a physical activities program.

BOREDOM. The occupational therapist who also acts as the recreational director is challenged by patient boredom. Patients/residents of a nursing home need diversion. The recreational director needs to find members of the nursing home who can help in this area. Any worker in the nursing home who has a talent should be encouraged to develop it for the benefit of the patients. Life within the walls of a nursing home soon becomes monotonous not only for the staff but also for the patient/resident. Variety can make life interesting and challenging. One should not forget the professionals who come in to work on the rehabilitation team; they too can contribute.

The occupational therapist is trained to evaluate through testing the perceptual reactions of a patient. Some simple tests are as follows:

1. The patient's ability to fit together a number of parts of a jigsaw puzzle.
2. The patient draws a picture of a bicycle or a house or person or automobile.
3. The patient has difficulty in positioning letters in writing.
4. The patient has some difficulty coping with directions or instructions.
5. The patient finds it difficult to dress self.

Tests must be used and the results considered when preparing a program for the patient. Finding perceptual defects is useful to the treatment plan by indicating that training must be broken down into simpler progressive steps than is common in the ordinary teaching process.

Occupational therapists are also trained to detect constructive apraxia, which is difficulty in assembling two-dimensional figures or patterns, such as arranging, building, and drawing with more than single movements. Tests that can be used to ascertain whether a patient has constructive apraxia are a paper and pencil test to copy designs and sticks of different lengths to duplicate a design demonstrated by the tester. The patient is asked to watch the tester closely and repeat the design demonstrated. If the patient crowds everything into one corner, he has constructive apraxia.

VISUAL AGNOSIA (mind blindness). Visual agnosia occurs in apperceptive and associational forms. A person with associational agnosia can copy a drawing but cannot identify it. A person with apperceptive agnosia is unable to draw a viewed object.

SPLINTS. The occupational therapist has been trained to improvise the making of splints. There are two types of splints that are made: (1) a resting splint, which helps in controlling pain, and (2) a corrective splint to reduce or retard deformity.

The methods and materials used for splints are many, but the most popular ones are (1) plaster of paris and (2) plastic with straps. Plastics that are often used are orthoplast and isoprene. These can be molded to a body part, if heated to a temperature of 140° F in a water bath. Royalite® must be heated on an electric hot plate to 300° F to be shaped but cannot be molded to a body part. Some plastics are softened with an organic solvent and hardens into the desired shape. Another type of splint is the Static Splint®, which is used to immoblize a part of the body that has experienced a fracture, inflammation, or operational procedure. In most cases, persons in a nursing home will come to the home with their own splints as ordered by their physicians.

Staff workers can and should understand the purposes of splints, and the occupational therapists can advise them. In splinting for the hands, fingers, and wrist, it is primarily the occupational therapist who has made significant contribution to the field of rehabilitation. Some indications for splints follow.

Splints are used primarily where the hand or wrist is involved in joint disease and muscle weakness, such as the patient with arthritis in his hands or the hemiplegic patient. If one of the upper extremities has weakness, the hand should be supported in a resting splint in a neutral position. This type of splint should be made of rigid, easy to clean material to protect the part. Stroke patients will often drop food on the involved part.

Rarely does the nursing home have a quadreplegic, and seldom do they have an amputee with a prosthesis for which the patient needs splints. But, if an occupational therapist is available, he is trained in these areas and could handle the situation.

CONCLUSION. Occupational therapists are an asset to any nursing home because of their educational background and knowledge. They fit in as part of the rehabilitation team, or they can work alone as an occupational therapist or a recreational director. They are a source of information to help and guide the staff worker.

As one studies the work of the occupational therapist, one must assume that the term occupational is not related to a person's vocational pursuit but means getting patients to occupy their time. The word work is used in conjuction with activities by a human being. Work is not necessarily something that is done by the personnel of the nursing home. Patients also must work to develop their physical strength, coordination, dexterity, and independence. Development of these characteristics are dependent upon what is available in the nursing home to improve them.

SPEECH AND HEARING

Speech and hearing is the foundation of communication. We send messages by speech, and we receive them through hearing. To understand, one must first receive information by sight or touch. Often nursing home staff members speak to patients, and they do not respond. This could be because they do not understand, but in many cases the reason was lack of hearing. The person who has probem hearing is hurt socially and educationally. In many cases, a hearing loss also produces some emotional problems.

Hearing loss may be conductive or neural or a mixture of the two. Conductive deafness usually results from some obstruction in the external or middle ear, which prevents auditory signals from reaching the brain through the inner ear. Perceptive hearing loss results from a lesion in the auditory complex of the inner ear.

It is interesting to note that the patient's family will most often notice that there is a hearing problem although the patient very rarely will admit that he has a problem. Usually, the family or staff physician will ask for a consultation with a specialist on this problem.

Better understanding of hearing problems will help the elderly patient and the staff workers who come in daily contact with them.

There is little one can do for a large percentage of people who have a hearing loss. There are some tests that can be used, however: (1) tuning fork, (2) pure tone audiometric, and (3) speech reception audiometric. Hearing is measured by determining the intensity in decibles of a so-called pure tone at various frequencies necessary to get a response from the patient under study.

There are three types of hearing losses:

1. Conductive hearing loss is due to a lesion in the external or middle ear.
2. Sensorineural hearing loss results from disease or injury, producing a lesion in the inner ear or along the auditory neural pathways.
3. Mixed hearing loss is a combination of both the preceding. Some of the causes of hearing loss are hereditary, and some are of toxic origin.

There are seven main causes for the three types of hearing losses:

1. Brain conditions
2. General infection diseases
3. Infections of the ear
4. Physical agents
5. Toxic agents
6. Miscellaneous
7. Advancing years

In rehabilitation, there are areas where the speech and hearing therapist can be of help. One area is in auditory training. If a person is learning to use a hearing aid, he needs help for period of time to learn how to use it properly. The length of time he will need assistance is variable, since some take more time than others.

Another method that is gaining in importance is speech reading, or lipreading. Speech is made up of vowel and consonant sounds. Speech reading is particularly valuable to adults because they lose their hearing for high frequencies. Deafness has a very profound psychologic effect on patients. It leads to paranoia, depression, hysteria, and suspiciousness on the part of patients.

A staff worker can help by telling the patient to accept that he has a hearing loss and to admit it openly. Once he has admitted this to himself, he can do a number of things to help the situation. He may ask a person to speak louder, learn to lip-read, or get a hearing aid.

One very important element in rehabilitation is to point out to the patient that in many cases there is nothing he can do about his deafness except accept it and follow the three steps mentioned previously. The person who is hard of hearing or who gradually has a loss of hearing is confronted by several problems. The general public assumes he is deaf and tries to communicate in other ways. The people with whom they are associated may have little patience with a person who has a hearing problem. The deaf need to learn to receive communications through channels other than hearing, as well as to develop means of self-expression.

PSYCHOLOGICAL IMPACT

Introduction

A patient who suffers a physical disability will at the same time suffer a psychological change. One of the problems of rehabilitation is that the physician treats only the organic disability, which the patient accepts and then waits for the miraculous cure. The rehabilitation team and the professionals in the field realize that patients must cooperate and be active in participating in their recovery. They cannot be passive and expect someone to do everything for them.

The Disability

Individuals develop a disability, i.e. a stroke or fracture of a hip. This crisis alters or changes a person's sensory, physical and psychological responses. They develop fears and doubts about survival, and in addition, they have new bodily sensations. They may have marked changes in sense of position of the body during movements. Furthermore, patients now find themselves in a new environment such as a hospital or nursing home. All of these factors make for disorganization in people's minds. How do they respond? Some patients rise to the new circumstances as a challenge, others become withdrawn and create problems for themselves, for their physicians, for their families, and for the professionals who want to rehabilitate them.

One of the main problems that confronts patients is the people surrounding them. The families of suddenly disabled members are appalled by the persons' disabilities. They think that loved ones will never recover and that they will have to do everything for them. They convey this feeling to the patients, who reacts by doing nothing and letting their families do for them. Then their families send them to a nursing home, and they are shocked by a new environment, where the staff expects patients to try to do things for themselves. All of these factors place a strain on the mental processes of patients.

Adjustment to a Handicap

For most patients who get a severe disability, there is a period of grief over their handicap, plus a period of time that they are plainly disorganized. They have profound fears of the future. Many think they will not be able to cope. They do not know what is possible in rehabilitating their disabilities, so they tend to underestimate what they will be able to accomplish. They start to compare themselves with others and, in doing so, arrive at negative thoughts. It is important that the people surrounding these patients do not overtly grieve for them and thus convey a feeling of hopelessness to them. A positive outlook will speed their rehabilitation. The staff members, the family, and the patients can start by looking at things that they can do today that they could not do yesterday. They will be encouraged by the improvements they discover in themselves. Once they have begun to discover some assets to their disabilities, they can be put into a nursing home to work toward rehabilitation. They soon take advantage of the professional team that surrounds them and start to develop both physically and mentally.

What about those patients and those families that have not accepted handicapped family members and their disabilities? In many cases families or spouses try to do too much for patients because it is easier to do for them than to watch them struggle to do things for themselves. On the other hand, if their families reject them or pay them no attention, they make exaggerated pleas for help in order to get some attention. These are two opposite reactions that influence the behavior of a disabled person.

In rehabilitation, it is the business of the staff to help the patients in their behavioral patterns. It is the administrator's business to cause behavioral patterns to change due to the settings or environment. Behavioral goals, in many cases, need to be either maintained or improved. It is important to recognize what the goals are for beneficial behavior to occur with appropriate frequency in the nursing home environment. For example, the goal of an elderly hemiplegic patient may be greater independence in self-care. Yet, what does this independence consist of in the nursing home? Is it the ability to get a hemiplegic patient to put on and to button his shirt when a physical therapist is watching him? It is quite important to have a program set up so that patients will do the same thing when they are alone. Thus, one must remember that the teaching-learning process is all-important in behavioral changes. Moreover, the criteria of effective learning should be for the behavior to occur wherever and whenever it is needed.

The Family

Patient's actions will be influenced to a large extent by the attitude of their families. If the families respond in ways that do not contribute to patient performance, patients will suffer accordingly. Patients will continue to improve if their families encourage them. Families need to learn a new image concerning the patients and a new set of values to help them develop new functional achievements. Thus, it is important to provide for systematic and repeated family participation in certain aspects of patients' programs. The professionals, like the social worker, recreational director, physical therapist, and others, must all work with the family. If possible, get them involved in planning activities for the patient outside the nursing home. Ascertain from them any problems that arise as a result of these excursions so that they can be solved as part of the patient's program.

Social Services

Many workers in nursing homes neglect to take into consideration that the patients they are treating may some day go home and back to their communities. It is true that not many patients, once they enter a nursing home, ever leave except to go back to the hospital or to visit somewhere for the day. However, many do cherish the thought that they could go home, and this can act as a powerful stimulus for rehabilitation. The will to achieve can be nourished and for those people who dream about going home, about putting this injury and illness in the past.

Social workers have a definite place on the rehabilitation team in most nursing homes. In most nursing homes, however, social workers are not part of the staff. Usually, they are representatives of a community agency or a welfare or family service. Social workers assume the leading role in preparing patients to return to home, family, and community. It would be helpful if social workers were involved with the rehabilitation team from the moment patients enter the nursing home until they leave.

The following are three areas in which the social worker can make valuable contributions:

1. Evaluation
2. Assistance in location of available social services
3. Consultation

In evaluation, they can bring to the attention of the physician and the rehabilitation team some factors that may influence the patient to cooperate with the staff, including (1) the strength and limitations of individuals seen in their behavior, (2) the family, peer, and cultural values, and (3) community services available. In making their evaluations, social workers consider patients' background to be important:

1. Physical description of patients
2. Social background
   a. Interests
   b. Vocational and recreational aims before disability
   c. Peer relationships — their nature and social role before disability.
3. Educational background, interest in education; amount of formal education
4. Family position
   a. Family structure; occupations and nature of the role of the family
   b. Family goals for the patient
   c. Family values and goals
   d. Family's reaction to patient's disability
   e. Family's reaction to patient's friends and to each other
   f. Family background; cultural, educational, socioeconomic

5. Patient's reaction to disability
6. Patient's expectation from the rehabilitative program
7. Patient's own goals and self-image
8. Patient's present relationship with family and with peers

The social worker is equipped to give this information to the family and to the patient.

The importance of patients' backgrounds in a total rehabilitation program cannot be emphasized too highly. The response of patients to medical treatment might be influenced by the attitudes, roles, and economics of their families and also by patients' ages and former occupations. The necessity for interviews with patients and their families are dependent upon the patients' responses to rehabilitation plans. Patients may not derive sufficient motiviation from their families, thus, they need other sources for encouragement. Social workers may unearth factors that have lain dormant for many years which may point to areas of current or anticipated trouble spots in the emotional and social relationships of the patient. If social workers know the attitudes of patients, they can help the nursing staff apply this knowledge to their approach in rehabilitation.

Social workers may limit their roles, in many cases, to consultations with the nursing home staff, or they may be extended to the planning and direction of a specific program.

Consultations

Consultations may be established on a variety of levels and often are dependent upon the relationship between all staff members. The most productive and effective method is the interdisciplinary conference, which includes the patient. This method requires a team relationship that has clearly defined roles for each of its members. The members of the team meet with the patient, who has the opportunity to direct questions to the team and to participate in the conclusions, which bring an answer to his questions. This type of meeting sometimes requires a preconference between the members to share information about the patient and to alert each other to possible questions that might be raised by the patient. From past experiences, the patient finds support in this type of conference; he learns that the team and staff of the nursing home share concern for him and work together to help him.

Another method that has been used is bringing patients to a staff meeting where some have conferences with part of the team while others have individual conferences with a single staff member. In yet another method, the patient is informed that anytime he feels the need for counseling or a conference, upon request he can talk with one member of the team, who has been assigned to him.

The social worker has a unique position in the field of rehabilitation, especially in a nursing home. In most cases, a nursing home has a limited budget, and by necessity, its staff is limited. Social workers representing agencies, private or state, with whom the nursing home has no relationship can be used to help in the rehabilitation of patients, if they are asked. The staff worker or team members can recommend that patients be interviewed by a social worker because of the problems that confront them.

Many patients have doubts and anxieties about themselves and their relationships with others. This may upset them and result in a multitude of changes in their emotional lives. The staff sees these signs, are aware of the patient's concerns, and realize they have someone to whom they can refer these patients.

On some occasions, the referral to social service is made at the time of an emotional crisis, when the patient's stress is intense and disruptive to medical treatment. This initiation of social service treatment at times of crisis may bring about immediate, but temporary, relief. The social worker may, after several interviews with the patient, affect the situation and diminish the extent of the patient's fears. However, a more favorable resolution of the patient's concerns may require a longer treatment program.

The belief that people can be quickly changed to adjust to a strange environment assumes that, like a prescription for eyeglasses to overcome a visual defect, it is a one time intervention. In reality, the concerned staff must look for the roots of the conflct and try to understand the nature of the problem. The social workers are sensitive; they listen to many sources around the patient and try to evaluate the problem to determine which part needs immediate assistance and which part gives patients their strength. In many cases, people who are unable to deal with their conflicts and problems may try to defend themselves against what appears to be a verbal attack.

Social service counseling is based on several judgments:

1. The nature and extent of the conflict.
   a. Tension may reflect repressed anxiety and a weak ego.
   b. It may also reflect clear perception of community attitudes and family disruptions.
2. Urgency of social work attention.
   a. How important are the problems that confront this patient?
   b. Do they interfere with his rehabilitation?
3. Does the patient recognize the problems?
4. The patient must recognize his weak and strong points. These need to be studied, and the patient must be guided into the proper channels to use his recognized strong points.

The social worker and the patient can focus on several levels. The nature of the conflct and the patient's strength may be such that he needs intensive counseling. The objectives of the counseling may be to help the patient seek answers to his conflicts and develop controls to handle new ones.

Patients Who Are About to Leave the Nursing Home

The transition from nursing home to other environment can be traumatic. The threat of failure is especially acute. The program and the shelter of the nursing home has been a comfort for patients. Any change of this environment dissolves this security, offering instead the unknown, which may build up tremendous fears. Transition from the home could mean a loss of social contacts that have become part of the patient's life.

The interval between nursing home and leaving to go back to the home and the community is heavy with tensions and could upset some patients to such an extent that they will refuse to leave. If they are left on their own after returning home, patients may flounder and fall back to become the responsibility of their communities. In many cases, they will not return to the nursing home for further assistance.

To minimize failure, which may once more impose inadequacy and isolation, the rehabilitation program must include a follow-up for a period of time after the individual has left the nursing home.

This phase must and can only be done by social workers. They must continue counseling and referral to community resources until the former patient has achieved the goals of rehabilitation and feels secure in his new environment. Social workers' plans should start long before the patient is ready for discharge.

The plan should reflect the rehabilitation team's consideration of the patient's physical, social, and psychological needs and the methods for further rehabilitation. The rehabilitation program may call for nursing care or physical therapy in the home. The plan should be studied and discussed with the patient and his family. Discharge plans should be part of the on-going interviews between the social worker, the patient, and the family so that the date and final decision will not impose a hasty departure.

SOCIAL WORKER

Social workers are trained in medical social work and are qualified to deal with the disabled through education and experience. They learn to develop attitudes that help others face and adjust to reality. Social work services can be defined as direct services to patients and their families. These services can be individual case work or group work or community organization. Case work includes (1) adjustment to environment changes and (2) psychological support.

Social workers seek to resolve personal and interpersonal relationships that stand in the way of a normal return of patients to home and community. Social workers will sometimes come into a nursing home and organize group work and activities. Their purpose is to help restore patients' abilities to participate, to react, and to derive support from others, especially in group recreation such as crafts, where services to others may be carried through successfully. Patients feel rewarded that they were able to help others more severely handicapped or disabled than they. Competent social workers give guidance to patients who are independent and want to return to community and home. They see that patients have places to live, either in their own homes or with families that want them. The economics of everyday living is looked into, and patients are given guidance in that area. If patients are still dependent and need a nurse, aide, or therapist to come into their own homes for a period of time, social workers take care of this. In short, they make a smooth transition from the nursing home to the patients' home and communities.

Social workers may use the interview approach or may find that a small group may be the most beneficial for the patients concerned. Each method has specific advantages, and the choice lies with the patients.

Individual Interviews

The interview approach affords patients and social workers the opportunity to develop the trust needed to discuss very intimate and conflicting problems. It permits such thoughts to emerge at a pace set by the patients, a pace that allows for emotional and intellectual development. The interview may be used to help patients to explore their conflicts, their goals, and their responses to certain situations. This is pointed out to disabled patients who assume a dependent role, who manipulate people to do things for them, or who argue with the therapists who are trying to get them to be independent. The interview can be used to help patients recognize that their response to people often brings about conflicts and shows them how they can change their attitude to their advantage.

The interview in many cases gives patients a feeling of importance. Patients who have fears and feel threatened by the other patients can look forward to the interview as a status symbol. They use this period as a time to tell their fears and apprehensions without fear of reprisals. They can test their behavior on the social worker to see what kind of response they get. This freedom of emotional expression may stimulate further social discourse.

Furthermore, during this period patients have time to think, to explore, to argue; they are not under pressure from other patients and strangers. They learn that the social worker will respond to their ideas. They develop and make decisions, which were difficult to arrive at before the interview.

Interview Setting

Usually patients are taken into an office set aside for interviews, if there is a visiting social worker. The office provides privacy. However, patients who are fearful and not accustomed to interviews might be benefitted by going to the dining room for a cup of coffee. Bed patients must be interviewed in their rooms, alone. Social workers must decide upon the locale depending on the particular patient. They must decide the time and the place appropriate for each interview.

Social workers have access to many other people to gather information, such as the doctor, the family, staff workers, and the rehabilitation team. All of this information can be brought back to patients in their interviews. They can bring a knowledge of the many facets of requirements made on patients by each of the people concerned. To patients, social workers may appear as top-ranked officials who use the interview to help them learn to participate in the many activities of the nursing home.

Social workers make home visits to gain specific information by talking to families. Many family members will not come to an office to discuss a patient's problems. The home visit also provides clues that cannot be given by descriptions offered across a desk. The family pattern of interaction can be observed and attitudes judged in the casual setting of the home. It is very important to have an accurate understanding of the family's reactions, values, and goals, as these assist or limit the patient's rehabilitation goals. Another reason for making a home visit is to meet families who do not come to the nursing home. This may be due to economics, fears, or indifference.

Group Interviews or Sessions

The group is recognized as a way to bring about interpersonal action needed to help the growth of individuals. The values of group work to rehabilitation are the following:

1. Education and support. Members of a group can share their problems and discover that others face the same crisis. Patients can relate their own attempts to deal with their problems and in doing so teach other group members how they may solve their situations.
2. Motivation. When people believe that they are alone, it breeds apathy and disillusionment. Personal contact can be helpful. Speaking to a group member who has gone through a similar

crisis or who is ahead in the rehabilitation process can encourage new attitudes. Sometimes contact between two members may provide motivation for the less disabled individual who gains reassurance of his strengths by comparison with the limitations of the other patient.

3. Socialization. Personality development is a continuing process. Social work with groups enhances the opportunities for continued growth in the process that comes from socialization. One level of participation allows patients to attend a group and sit quietly listening to others. This quiet participation allows patients to gain support by hearing the experiences of others without having to confront these conflicts. Being present is what is important. They learn something about the behavior of others and relate this to their problems.

The social worker may introduce experiences with opportunity for achievement, and as patients gains status, they can relate more intimately with peers. The individual, by means of social activities, can test his social strengths and become aware of social interactions and challenge others, thereby encouraging development of accurate social perception.

A good group leader has a specific role; he sets the stage so that certain experiences are planned and achieved. He brings specific ideas and thoughts to the group, thereby provoking interaction. He focuses on individual responses to get supporting or conflicting expressions. He gives them direction so that as a group they learn to handle new experiences. The group meeting is a setting in which social life develops.

The methods used by a social worker vary in order to relate to each patient's age, social abilities, intellectual abilities, recreational interests, needs, and rehabilitation goals. Some use arts and crafts or specific games or music or other activities.

Social Services Available

Some communities have health and welfare directories that list the types of social services offered:

1. Public assistance: Social Security Act.

2. Public assistance programs: Contributions from federal and state agencies.
3. Old age assistance (OAA): Gives aid for people over sixty-five years of age.
4. Aid to the blind.
5. Permanently disabled.
6. Family service agencies.
7. Settlement house, community centers, Y.M.C.A., Y.W.C.A.
8. Community public health or mental health programs.
9. Universities with schools of social work.

NURSING SERVICE

Nursing is concerned with physical, social, and emotional functioning of patients. All members of the nursing service must be made aware of their responsibilities. The nursing service staff includes the head nurse or the director of nursing, the charge nurse, general duty nurses, licensed vocational nurse (L.V.N.), the licensed practical nurse (L.P.N.), and the nurses' aides. Usually, working on the same level of administration as the director of nursing is the head dietitian, the physical therapist and/or occupational therapist, the social worker, and the recreational or activities director.

Nursing service is part of the rehabilitation team that works together for the best interests of patients. Since a nursing home has as one of its objectives the rehabilitation of its patients, the director of nursing must be made cognizant of the field of rehabilitative nursing. In addition to their normal functions, they must learn the techniques of rehabilitation and be aware of emotional factors related to physical disability. Part of their training will be understanding problems peculiar to various disabilities methods by which disabled persons use remaining muscular function, measures for preventing further disability, treatment of existing disabilities, and improvement of communication skills. Soon they learn from practical experiences or from other professionals in specialized fields that there is a need for providing preventive and therapeutic nursing therapies. Teaching patients and families preventive and self-care activities in keeping with the patients' abilities and integrating the contributions of various professionals into the patients' program on a twenty-four hour basis is part of the nursing staff's responsibility. If the director of nursing does a good job, the rehabilitation team should accomplish its goals efficiently.

Nursing service includes all the things the nurse does for and with the patient that are not necessarily ordered by the physician or by another professional from the team or staff. This covers meeting the physical needs of patients such as food, comfort, cleanliness, skin care, and elimination, helping patients to help themselves, providing emotional support, being attentive to needs, and getting them to interact with persons in their environment.

The nursing director is responsible for teaching and supervision of all nursing staff who are in contact with patients. Teaching can be considered working with patients to demonstrate activities for the auxiliary staff to do. Teaching is also having in-service training for the staff who work with the patients. It is most successful if there is a scheduled time for these teaching periods.

Nurses who go into the field of rehabilitation nursing have a difficult time adjusting the priorities in their thinking. In rehabilitative nursing, the aim is teaching them to do for themselves, meaning the patients. In regular nursing, emphasis is on doing for the patient, so this is quite a new concept. In fact, this involves quite a change in a person's training and thinking. The nursing service approach is the foundation for the rehabilitative process. It is an educational process in which the future of patients depends on the learning and growth that takes place during the treatment and care of in the facility. At the first meeting with patients, the nursing staff becomes aware of their physical aspects. They must prevent physical disability because this shortens treatment time. This includes maintaining joint mobility, good skin care, and cleanliness. Teaching self-care activities promotes physical function. Teaching patients safe and efficient functioning allows them to use their energy in more positive ways. If independent function can be achieved, it is the key to all activities that the patients are taught. The nurse first looks at the patient, then listens to the patient's verbal responses, which supply the ideas that determine the nurse's behavior toward the patient.

Patients' emotional behavior patterns — withdrawal, dependency, regression, and aggression — have already been discussed. The reason for these symptoms was enforced dependency as a result of the disability. Much can be said about allowing the patient to release his aggression and anxiety by exploding his anger and listening to him. The nurse becomes a person providing comfort and support while patients are making adjustments to function in their new environment. The nurses start a new interaction with patients who will be with them for various lengths of time.

The physical setting is most important to this new relationship. If there is a stimulating atmosphere, this encourages the patients to participate in activities that contribute to their mental, as well as physical, health. If there is interaction, then there is the needed socialization, which is best carried out in social functions such as coffee time and other activities. This prevents people who are withdrawn from being inactive. Arrangements should be made to allow privacy in meetings between family and patient. Nurses may sit in at these meetings to get guidance in the care of the patient by input from the family.

How do nurses work? They too develop their programs for a patient by gathering information. They first examine a patient, observing physical condition, skin condition, range of motion of joints, involuntary muscle movements, and any indications of emotional, psychological, and social needs. They talk to families to get relevant facts. The physician gives the diagnosis, evaluation, and suggestions for any limitations in activities, plus orders for medications. Then there will be reports and observations from other specialists such as social worker, physical therapist, dietitian, and others in nursing service.

Nurses and Their Treatment Plan

The director of nursing has in hand the reports from all nursing staff as well as from other professionals on the team. For example, the director has the physical therapist's reports on the patient's physical capacity and limitations, the patient's needs in this field, a suggested program with immediate objectives and goals, and long-range objectives and goals.

With all of these reports in hand, the director of nursing talks to the patient, listening and learning how to relate to the patient's disability. The director contacts the family and learns about the patient's background — how the patient relates to his family and to other patients and what his social and economic background is.

Then the director calls a conference and discusses a tentative schedule for a week or a month, whichever is indicated. This plan must be flexible; it might be changed daily at first, as new facts about the patient are learned. Is the patient comfortable with the program? Is he responding to the treatment? What are his reactions? Are there any changes in the patient physically or mentally? Is he eating well? Has his socialization revealed any indications of his reactions to the facility? Changes in the program are needed as the patient progresses.

If nursing service is to do a good job, there must be a good system of communication between all members of the nursing service and other members of the rehabilitation team. Verbal communication and written reports should be done almost daily to ensure that the plan of treatment is carried out on a twenty-four-hour basis, in the most efficient manner.

This early treatment plan must be adjustable. It must allow for more time for some activities and less for those that change in a short time. Priorities must be set up. For example, if the patient has a bowel problem, his time in physical therapy might be cut until this condition is improved. Coordination through a schedule of activities should consider the patient's needs as well as his choices.

Each member of the team must make adjustments in its goals as the patient's condition changes. The treatment plan must include not only the physical but the emotional, the social, and recreational aspects of rehabilitation. Nursing service members coordinate all aspects of the treatment plan. They are second in command to the physician. They must do all the arranging for all aspects of a patient's needs.

The nurse is responsible for the medical orders that are given by the physician, such as changing dressings, checking indwelling catheters, and administering medications. In many cases, if there is no physical therapist, the nurse must carry on the activities that were started in the hospital, such routine activities as helping with range of motion exercises, supervising the new ambulatory patient, giving special exercises, and checking on the use of special devices that the patient needs. Many activities that the physical therapist would do are done by a nurse trained in rehabilitation. The nurse take over many of the duties of the specialists that compose a rehabilitation team.

As the patient improves, the treatment program becomes one of guidance to new and more advanced activities. If there are not consultants, the nurse must be the sole judge in determining needed changes, unless the physician will advise on patient care.

In deciding about an activity, one must take into consideration the patient's —

1. muscle function;
2. muscle tightness;
3. trunk balance;
4. limitation of R.O.M.;
5. endurance;
6. mental abilities;
7. emotional readiness.

After considering these factors, the nurse discusses any indicated changes in the treatment plan with the patient. Many new functions and activities are not formalized treatment periods but are done in conjunction with everyday routine. For example, teaching activities of daily living are done in the room, dressing, combing hair, going to the bathroom, etc. They can and should be taught at the appropriate time and as soon as feasible. The same applies to transfer techniques, such as getting in and out of wheelchairs. These activities can best be done in nursing homes by knowledgeable nurses and the staff.

Equipment

One of the aids to nursing service to help carry out its function in rehabilitation is the use of proper equipment. In many cases, workers in rehabilitation expend a lot of energy working with the handicapped patient. One way of conserving this energy is using proper equipment.

The bed level should be high if patients are full-time bed patients and low if they are able to get out of bed without help. The height of the bed must be suitable for nursing staff to render the best service. It helps the staff worker if the bed is electric. The mattress should be firm so that the sheets do not wrinkle and irritate the skin of the patient. Side rails for safety should be part of the bed. There should be stops on the casters of the bed so it does not roll while trying to get the patient in or out of bed. Many patients can use an overhead trapeze as part of their rehabilitation exercises. Finally, a footboard should be part of the equipment to prevent drop foot and to carry the weight of the covers.

Additional Functions of the Nurse

Earlier in the discussion of the functions of the nursing service, it was pointed out that one of the main nursing duties is taking care of the patient who is bedfast. The patient must not be allowed to get contractures, muscular atrophy, or bed sores. Exercises must be carried out properly to prevent the development of these conditions. If the physician does not contraindicate exercises, the nursing service must carry out this function. The nurse needs to know the patient's range of motion, loss of muscular function that can cause tightness, and the degree of sensation. If a patient has a fracture, the physician will indicate the best position for that patient.

Positioning

Observation is one of the keys for people who want to help a handicapped patient. They must observe a patient's bodily segments and the position they assume when sitting, standing, or lying in bed. They must note the skin condition, such as dryness, irritation, breaks, and redness, check prominent pressure joints to prevent pressure sores, and be aware of involuntary movements.

The footboard that aids in positioning has been mentioned. The use of rolled towels or sheets, foam rubber pads, and a variety of sizes of pillows and sandbags, properly placed, will prevent the formation of contractures and keep the patient properly positioned. For example, to keep the lower extremity upright and not rotated laterally, a towel roll is extended from the knee to the trochanter under the lateral side of the thigh. Especially for people with a stroke, a small pillow at the neck on the involved side will prevent contracture of the neck and keep the head straight; a sandbag can be used to keep a leg and foot upright. Some patients will benefit from the use of a water mattress, especially if they are heavy because it equalizes the weight distribution. Mention should be made of the saddle bag, which is a sandbag connected to another sandbag by straps or a piece of canvas so that it can be put across an arm or leg to keep it in place.

The patient who cannot or does not turn himself must have a positioning plan developed, which includes (1) time to change and (2) position variations.

To maintain joint mobility and good condition of the skin and to increase normal physiological processes, usually a change of position every two hours is indicated, with close observation for pressure areas. The time must be decreased if there is redness of the skin, soreness, or irritation. Some aids to help protect areas of bony prominences is the use of sheepskin or synthetic fiber around, but not over, the bony prominences. Some people need padding under their braces.

The position of the patient who is allowed out of bed to get into either a chair or wheelchair is very important. At first, the best thing to do is to allow the patient to become adjusted to this new sitting position and then let him get back to bed. For the proper positioning in a chair one must ask what segments of the patient's body need support, how erect can they sit, how long can they sit, and can they get in and out of bed with or without help? Will it be easier to teach them to get in and out of the chair first or will it be better for the patient to be lifted by the staff? These elements must be considered before any changes are made in the treatment plan of the patient.

As patients progress, the physician notes the changes, or the nurse brings it to his attention, and they go one step further into rehabilitation by starting active range of motion with or without resistance, muscle setting, isometric exercises, breathing, or other exercises aimed at the patient's handicap. One of the most effective forms of active exercises is performing the activities of daily living, sometimes called self-care activities, such as (1) moving in bed, (2) sitting up, (3) transferring, (4) dressing, and (5) maintaining personal hygiene. All of these may improve range of motion, strengthening muscles and developing coordination and balance.

There is a need to go into further detail concerning the ambulatory or nonambulatory patient who spends most of his time in bed. He needs to change positions, to get in and out of bed and chairs, to perform the activities of daily living, and to do other activities in bed such as turning and moving from one side of the bed to the other. It has been mentioned, but bears repeating, that a firm mattress is a great help to the patient who wants to move in bed. The method of moving depends upon the physical disability of the patient.

A patient who has unilateral involvement

1. Turning to the uninvolved side from the supine position:
    a. Support the involved hand on the chest.
    b. Place the heel of the strong leg over the ankle of the weak one.
    c. Flex the weak hip and knee by pulling with the heel of the strong leg and with the strong arm.
    d. Place the strong hand on the outer side of the knee, straighten the normal leg, and pull toward the strong side.
2. Turning to the involved side from the supine position:
    a. Flex strong hip and knee, grasp side rail with strong hand.
    b. Push up and over with the leg, and pull with the hand.
3. Moving in the prone position:
    a. Flex strong hip and knee.
    b. Push or pull with strong arm (patient will usually move toward his strong side).

For other changes of position, patients may use the side rails for leverage or a strap or knotted rope tied to the end of the bed or the trapeze, or they may push against the footboard.

A paraplegic who has both legs paralyzed but has strength in his arms can move by using his arms to bed his legs, then lean them in the direction he wants to turn, push on knees in that direction, and turn. These patients can use the trapeze for moving by lifting themselves. This gives them a pulling exercise. However, remember that to get in and out of bed and perform other transfers, the main muscles that need to be developed are the pushing muscles, the extensors. Push-ups, which will strengthen these muscles, should be a part of the patient's program.

Transferring Patients

The nursing service has one of its most important functions in transferring patients properly because this reduces the number of personnel involved, and the staff members do not hurt themselves by heavy lifting and carrying. Transferring is no problem if a mechanical lift is available and the staff knows how to use it. Some patients are able to shift, lift, and slide to position with very little help.

The basic method used for individuals, of course, depends on their condition. Since transferring is done so often during the day, it allows for a great deal of practice. The method used not only depends on the patient's condition, but the surface the patient is on and the surface they are transferring to.

The Mechanical Lift

The mechanical lift is used when patients cannot assist to a great extent. A stretcher or a sling that supports the patient in a full- or half-sitting position is used. A sling is needed if this patient will be put into a chair or wheelchair. There are lifts that permit patients to be put into car seats, which can be used to get patients out of, as well as into, a wheelchair or chair. The stationary type of lifts are used to put patients into a bathtub. Safety is the key to any method used for sitting or standing transfers.

Sitting Transfers

The person with one strong lower extremity usually can transfer better when moving that side of his body toward the chair or bed. For example, the patient with a left hemiplegia will move best towards his right side. If a person has involved muscular problems, like the arthritic, the stronger arm is used as a stabilizer during standing and pivoting. Some aids in transfers that are helpful for patients with poor or fair balance and physical disabilities is equalizing the height of the transfer surfaces. Supporting patients' feet on the floor and raising the height of the chair seat will increase their stability during sitting transfers. Throughout the whole transfer period, the helper must keep in mind that he is trying to teach patients to become independent. This is a golden opportunity to get them to participate as much as possible. Each time they are helped too much in a transfer, patients lose a chance to learn how to do this for themselves.

Force of Gravity

Gravity is an important force in transfers. It assists when lowering the body; it must be overcome when lifting the body. Putting the patient's legs off the bed will make them slide down to the floor, then he raises his trunk upward against the force of gravity to the sitting position. At first he may need help with the latter. Patients learn to do this by themselves next and learn trunk balance when sitting. First, the helper points out that the center of gravity of the trunk should be kept a little forward of the vertical position. Support of the arms when transferring is important. By placing them in front of the hips, with the near arm towards the transfer object and leaning the trunk slightly in the direction of movement, the center of gravity is shifted toward the transfer object, permitting the seat to slide laterally.

Standing Transfer

It is important to get the segments properly positioned so that patients can stand with the least effort (Fig. 8-9). By moving the head and trunk forward, the center of gravity is brought forward. All that is left to be done to stand is to move upward against gravity by extending the hips and knees. If necessary, patients may pull up on something such as a locked wheelchair or handrail. To transfer from standing to a sitting position, the patient will move toward the transfer object by pivoting on the stronger lower extremity. The stronger arm may be used as a stabilizer during the sitting phase, which entails controlling gravitational force, which is 32 feet per second.

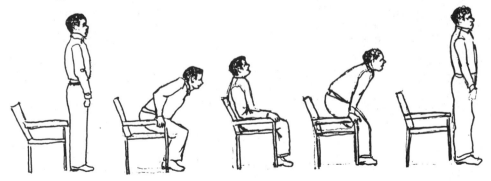

Figure 8-9. How to sit down and get up. The main points in sitting are starting with the calves against the chair, chin out in front, and hands placed firmly on arms of the chair to carry body weights. To get up, slide forward in the chair and basically do the sitting process in reverse.

Walking Patients

In cases where there is no physical therapist supervising the ambulation of these patients, the nurse takes over. The physician or this book will help teach how to measure crutches or a walker, if needed. The gait pattern will usually be the basic pattern of the two-or three-point gait, if the patient does not have a severe disability. Patients who are learning to walk or have learned a gait pattern need practice. The attendant giving ambulation practice should use a belt fastened around the patient's waist for safety if the patient is a beginner or if he is unstable or weak. If possible, the nursing home should have a physical therapy consultant to advise the nursing service.

There are various aids that the patient should use, depending upon his disability, such as —

1. short or long leg brace to support knee and ankle;
2. elastic bandages;
3. back braces;
4. binders for trunk alignment;
5. slings or splints.

The nursing service needs training in how to apply the devices and how to teach the patients to apply and use them. Many times they have to keep these pieces of equipment clean, oiled, and repaired to avoid a minor breakdown.

Wheelchair Patients

There are many patients who are able to sit but cannot stand. These people are then put in wheelchairs. Most of them use a standard chair, and there are no problems, except to see that the patient gets into the chair and out of it when he wants to go to bed. The patient should be comfortable. Usually a seat cushion adds comfort in sitting, and if the person is small, this gives them the needed height for other activities. Sometimes a back cushion is needed to give some support for the back and take the pressure off the lumbar-sacral area. Litter carriers are used by patients to carry things around with them, when going to another room, to the recreation area or any place that they may need some of their basic needs.

Pressure Sores (Bed Sores or Decubitus Ulcer)

The lack of mobility and movement in bed or wheelchairs cause pressure sores, which are a major problem for patients, regardless of disability, and are a vital impediment to the progress of rehabilitation. Pressure sores are the result of impaired blood supply to weight-bearing areas and bony prominences caused by pressure, which compresses arteriolar vessels to the extent that tissues become devitalized and subsequently slough off, many times to the underlying bony surfaces. The length of time for this to occur depends upon the degree of pressure and the ability of the person to shift his weight and to change positions.

The primary causes of these sores are disability, sedation, obesity, or emotionally induced inertia. Thus, one must continuously caution patients to move in order to maintain mobility. Of course, some patients are unable to move and will need help. Emphasis is on prevention. Once a pressure sore is present, it may take months for it to heal. Sometimes, as a last resort, radical surgery is performed. Signs or symptoms are (1) persistent redness, (2) breakdown of skin, and (3) sloughing of all devitalized tissue.

Prevention depends upon being on a constant lookout for early warning symptoms. Check areas of weight bearing — the sacral area in the supine position, the greater trochanteric region when sidelying. Also, check areas having bony prominences, as the heel, and lateral side of the ankle. Is there redness? If so, the patient should move and shift the weight-bearing areas; if the patient is unable to move, assign him to a staff member who should reposition him on a time schedule. Hopefully, the redness will disappear within twenty-four hours. If not, this is a problem. The area must be relieved of all pressure, either by discontinuing the position that caused the symptom or by bridging the area with the proper placement of supports, such as small compact pillows, rolls, rings, pad made of sheepskin or synthetic fiber, or doughnuts made of felt for small areas. Ingenuity helps here. Never put a pad under the red area; it only increases the pressure. When a breakdown of skin or sloughing are present with or without infection, a topical dressing must be applied while carrying out measures to relieve pressure. When positioning these patients, be doubly careful that pressure areas do not occur elsewhere.

To repeat, the key point in preventing pressure sores is to move. It is the responsibility of the nursing staff to help the patient by making sure there are timely changes of position. Some important points to remember are the following:

1. An ambulatory patient stays out of bed most of the time and moves around as much as possible.
2. Wheelchair-bound patients must be taught to relieve pressure every hour by doing wheelchair push-ups and by shifting weight in chair and in bed, especially at night.
3. If possible, the patient should learn to turn and move himself. After he learns this, they must do it by following a time schedule and a list of the positions to be done alone or with the help of a staff member.
4. As soon as the staff see a reddened area they must carry out the routine listed previously.
5. Try to distribute the pressure evenly over the entire body when in bed.
6. Sheets and dressings should be loose and soft; this might look bad when the patient is on an air mattress.

Useful Aids

1. Boots for prevention of sores on heels. This helps to keep the foot in the proper position regardless of the bodily position (Fig. 8-10).
2. For wheelchair patients a horseshoe-shaped pad on the seat of the chair to relieve pressure on the sacral area is useful.

SUMMARY OF THE KNOWLEDGE, SKILLS, AND ATTITUDES OF NURSE AND NURSING SERVICE

Rehabilitation nurses must develop a greater depth of knowledge, skills, and attitudes if they are to treat the aged, handicapped person in a nursing home in a successful manner. First, nurses need a good understanding of the psychological effects of long-term illness in order to respond appropriately to the patient's needs during the various stages of adjustment to a handicap. Furthermore, they must increase their knowledge of anatomy, physiology, the musculoskeletal system the science of movements, and kinesiology. Also, they should possess the ability to speak clearly and be understood by patients, family, and administration. The

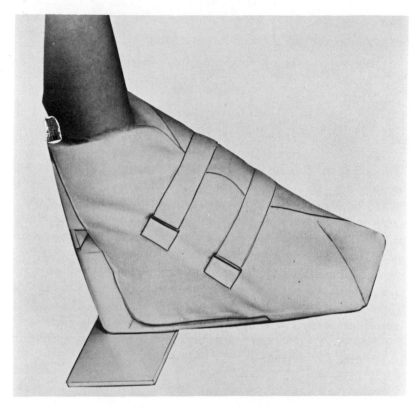

Figure 8-10. Boot for ankle.

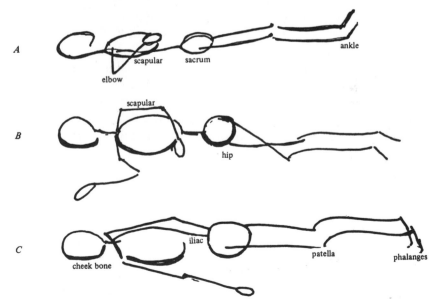

Figure 8-11. Bony prominences most vulnerable to pressure sores. A. Supine position. B. Side-lying position. C. Prone position.

following special skills have been discussed:

1. Positioning, to prevent deformities and to prevent pressure sores.
2. Transfer techniques
3. Range of motion exercises
4. Exercises, active, passive, and active assistance
5. Attitude

Good rehabilitative nurses must have patience and understanding so they can respond to their patients. They usually are slow geared because their elderly patients move at a slower pace. As sensitive people, they adjust their actions according to each patient. At certain times, patients may need a lot of encouragement and praise by the nurses will give the patients strength to carry on. Because improvement is so slow at times, praise for the patient's efforts is needed rather than for the improvement shown. Time and more time is what patients need; therefore, the teacher must have patience. Repetition is the key note to learning for the elderly and disabled. Patients must repeat and repeat and repeat until they learn to do a procedure automatically.

Learning and Relearning

How to dress, to walk, and to do the dozens of things needed in everyday living activities is a very slow process. Giving patients time to learn is the only way. This means allowing time for patients to do things for themselves. It is very difficult to refrain from assisting patients during these periods of learning. Sometimes nurses, in their haste, do too much for them; this simply undoes the preceding work.

The nursing service progress should move from simple to complex procedures. Patients make adjustments from home or hospital to the nursing home, and then maybe back home. In a nursing home, nurses are very much independent. In most instances, the physician will give them a free hand with patients except for strictly medical procedures. Nurses must do things as they see the need and not wait for orders.

The use of footboards, bedboards, turning shedules, positioning, range of motion exercises, comfort measures, and all other measures must be initiated by the nurses. They are on duty twenty-four hours a day, and these are their responsibilities.

The need for coordination between members of the rehabilitation team and the nursing director, who is the key person to see that rehabilitation is implemented, has been discussed. This means coordination of the expertise of various therapies into a patient's activities throughout the day. For example, if a patient spends thirty minutes once a week with the speech therapist, the patient will need to practice what was taught between his lesson periods. In order to do this, the nurse needs to know what the speech therapist wants the patient to practice. This information becomes part of the patient's program. The same holds true for all other therapies.

It is most important for nurses to have a good channel of communication with all the members of the team that work with the patient. The routine that is best is the one that accomplishes the most for the patient.

REFERENCES

1. *Handbook of Physical Therapy,* by Robert Shestack. Springer Publishing Co., New York City.
2. United States Department of Labor, Manpower Administration, *Dictionary of Occupational Titles,* Vol. 1 & 2. United States Government Printing Office, Washington, D.C., 1975.
3. *Manual of Physical Therapy,* by Richard Kovacs. Lea & Febiger Publishers, Philadelphia, 1949.
4. *Rehabilitation and Medicine,* by Sidney Licht. Waverly Press, Inc., Baltimore, 1968.
5. *Occupational Therapy in Rehabilitation,* by E.M. McDonald. Williams and Wilkins Co., Baltimore, 1976.
6. Ready for Geriatrics, by N. Johnson. *American Journal of Occupational Therapy, 19:*192, 1965.
7. The Efficiency of Instructions for Hemiplegic Patients, by W.A. Fordyce and R.H. Jones. *Archives of Physical Medicine, 47:*676, 1966,
8. *A Social Worker's Guide,* by G. Travis. Berekley Press, Berkeley, California, 1966.
9. *Physical Disability: A Psychological Approach,* by B.A. Wright. Harper & Row, New York, 1965.
10. *Encyclopedia of Social Work,* edited by John Turner. National Association of Social Workers, New York, 1977.
11. *The Rehabilitation Agency and Social Work,* by V.M. Seider and R. Stienman. United States Department of Health, Education and Welfare, Vocational Rehabilitation Administration, Washington, D.C., 1966.
12. *Rehabilitative Nursing Techniques,* by C.H. Coles. A procedure for Passive

Range of Motion and Self-Assistive Exercises. Kennedy Rehabilitation Insititute, Minneapolis, Minnesota, 1967.

13. *Handbook of Rehabilitative Nursing,* by American Rehabilitative Foundation. Techniques in Hemiplegia. Kennedy Rehabilitation Institute, Minneapolis, Minnesota, 1964.

14. The Nurse Therapist in a Rehabilitation Setting, by Nancy et al. *American Journal of Nursing, 70:*1694, 1970.

Chapter 9

PSYCHOSOCIAL ASPECTS OF
REHABILITATION

INTRODUCTION

IN the healthiest people there is some degree of mental problems, which may be because of memories, excess tension, worry, or fear. Research has demonstrated that sick minds and emotions of older persons are not caused by time. Instead they are the result of (1) situations affecting the aged, (2) disease, or (3) both of the preceding.

Physical and mental health are closely interrelated. There are a number of components of mental illness in nearly every physical illness. For example, most stroke victims have primarily physical effects — ones that are visible and obvious. Yet, after a person finds himself unable to move his body or to speak clearly the shock and frustration, if left untreated, may be as disturbing as the loss of physical control itself. Thus, he is doubly immobilized — physically and mentally.

Special emotional hazards are characteristic of aging. As people grow older they develop limitations of vision, hearing, physical dexterity, and endurance. They also experience difficulties with memory and coordination. Emotional problems of the aged are a little different from those of anyone else. Also, the emotional outlook and the psychological way of reacting to problems change with time. Thus, the early detection of a mental disturbance is extremely important.

In the treatment of an individual, one must remember at all times that the physical, the psychological, and the psychosocial aspects must be treated as a unit. The previous chapters have dealt with physical restoration of a disease or ailment. The staff of a nursing home and the professionals who see the patients every day must at all times be aware of the many problems that confront their patients. Thus, this chapter will deal with another phase of rehabilitation, the psychosocial.

297

EVALUATION

When the patient has been admitted and the diagnosis has been put on the chart by the physician, this takes care of the physical aspect, but the social aspects that might contribute to the success of the rehabilitation program, or lack of success if the social problems outweigh the physical problems, are not known. Thus, an important phase is an evaluation of the patient's social needs. A staff member who is interested in this aspect of rehabilitation should be assigned to patients to ascertain the following:

1. Information concerning patients' home life before their disabilities including economic conditions, family, interests, what they are going to do if discharged, and any other pertinent details.
2. The injury that affected the patients, their personalities, their family relationships, and their economic situations.
3. In case they are discharged, find out (a) who will assist them, (b) whether they will be in their home or apartment, (c) whether their families will help, (d) what the economic situation is.

The information must be gathered by many interviews with patient, family, relatives, and friends.

The staff members who are making this evaluation must be understanding and sympathetic; they must have patience and concern for people. They should be acquainted with the many local social agencies, the people who run these agencies, and the services they are willing to do for the people.

The aims of all the agencies must coincide with the aims of the patient. During the interviews with patients, the staff must try to ascertain the problems that are bothering the patient and, if possible, the solution. These problems might arise from the patient's physical ailment, from his anxieties, or from other emotional aspects that have arisen as a result of his handicap or because he left home to go to a nursing home.

TREATMENT

After making the evaluations, one should concentrate on methods of helping patients. All patients are different, yet each deserves the best treatment possible. Following is a list of types of people the staff will encounter.

1. The robust
2. The irrepressively optimistic extrovert
3. The withdrawn
4. The incorrigible defeatist
5. The introvert

Furthermore, there are as many variations within these types as there are people under the staff's care.

In many cases, the major physical disability has greatly affected the patient's minor disabilities. Psychologically, each one has contributed, and the staff should react accordingly. It is important to remember that every patient is affected psychologically by a physical disability.

The informal approach to ascertain a patient's needs and then to treat them accordingly is most strongly recommended for a nursing home. It is too expensive to obtain the services of a psychologist or psychiatrist for the psychological or psychosocial treatment of patients. The member of the staff who is most fit to study and help patients in this area is the head nurse. Nurses come in contact with the patient upon arrival. They are the ones who read and understand the patient's charts. They have direct communication with the patients' physicians. The family of the patient looks to the nurses for guidance and help. Nurses are the ones who give directions to the staff for the welfare of the patient. They try to make the patient feel safe and comfortable in his new surrounding. They are the ones in whom the patient confides. Nurses can modify any rules for the welfare of the patient. For example, if the patient is worried about some condition at home, the nurse can make the phone call or arrange to have the patient make the call to relieve the patient of his anxieties.

Patients are encouraged to feel that someone cares for them in this new environment. It is essential that the patients be convinced that the staff is there to help them get well, and if they so desire, they can go home. In addition to the head nurse's regular duties, it is important to do any psychosocial work that is necessary. The nurse must work closely with the social worker or workers of different agencies that are available, to help when and if the patient is ready for discharge. Therefore, we must look into the role of the social worker.

DISCHARGE

The responsibility for determining the eligibility for discharge of a patient from a nursing home lies directly with the head nurse or nursing director after consultation with the physician in charge of that patient. However, it is the social worker who must coordinate all of the findings made by the nurse during the patient's stay in the nursing home with the data provided by the family and the community relating to family resources, financial status, opportunity to resume normal roles of work, and any other details important to the welfare of the patient. The availability of programs for financial assistance, if needed, continuing social services, and medical checkups should be investigated.

At this point, it is safe to say that many nursing homes make no plans for patients after they leave the nursing home. In fact, they do not consider that patients will ever leave the nursing home once they are brought there. Thus, if patients do get well and go home, frequently due to no planning or poor planning with no social worker involved, patients return to the nursing home in far worse condition, physically and mentally, to spend the rest of their days there. To avoid this, a brief outline of the work of a social worker has been included to acquaint the staff of a nursing home with the many pitfalls that may be encountered by patients who leave the nursing home without proper preparations for their return to the community.

FACTOR INFLUENCING PSYCHOSOCIAL REHABILITATION

Does the patient want to get well? Does the patient have something to work for — a goal or objective? Factors to be studied for rehabilitation are (1) physical condition, (2) mental attitudes, and (3) emotional stability. If the patient is superior in these three characteristics, then the chance of recovery is high. If inferior, then there is less likelihood of recovery. The mental outlook is one of the most important aspects of rehabilitation. If people have physical deficiencies but are motivated, they can be helped by various devices and methods. However, if they have a mental impairment, it is very difficult, and sometimes impossible to do anything for them.

Such factors as fear, uncertainty, depression, and withdrawal must be considered. In addition, if the medical staff or nursing staff give thoughtless, inadequate, or noncommunicative attention to the patient, it is detrimental to the patient. Urging patients to do things for themselves immediately after their illness starts a chain reaction antagonistic to their recovery.

To integrate the patient as a member of the rehabilitation team, some important, seemingly minor things can be done:

1. Allow them to wear their own nightclothes.
2. Let them retain some of their personal possessions.
3. Promote self-care.
4. Provide opportunity for self-expression.
5. Allow participation in decisions concerning their treatment.

PSYCHOMOTOR RESPONSES

A simple way of explaining psychomotor responses is to give an example. If a person has new sensory input (information), this new information through perceptual and integrative processes determines whether there is need for any action. Instructions are then sent to the appropriate activity center (a muscle) to activate responses. If there is a handicap, then this chain reaction would be limited where weakness or handicaps exist. It could be limited by changes in sensory perception, the transmission from perception to action, or the strength of the sensory signal and muscular output.

Psychomotor performances change as an individual ages. Reaction time increases with age. But, reaction time can, will, and does become affected by motivation. It is also important to remember that the nature of the stimulus and the complexity of the response will affect reaction time. The aged will show slower speed of movement. Precision of response also declines with age. In many cases, the elderly will take more time to be more exact or accurate. Age decrements in performance seem to relate to cerebral cortex functioning rather than to any loss of ability to move. Circulatory deterioration, reduced cerebral metabolism, and/or suppressed brain rhythms tend to produce slower reaction time.

Cardiovascular problems may also serve to depress reaction time in a way that cannot be overcome by exercise. In psychomotor performances, the decline is seen often in the social functioning of an individual. Jobs that were formerly no problem, such as driving a car or operating a lawn mower, may become a problem as a result of advancing years. Some activities that are directly related to a person's health may become more difficult to carry out. The nature and decline of psychomotor performance is such that it is difficult to offset them mechanically in the same way that glasses or hearing aids can be used to offset the decline in sensory perception.

INTELLIGENCE

There is no definite proof that with age comes a lessening of intelligence. Measurement of intelligence is a highly controversial subject. It is safe to say that if people are tested on subjects that have no relationship to their present or past experiences, they would make a low score. On the other hand, when elderly persons were tested against younger people on (1) use of the telephone, (2) common legal terms, or (3) social security benefits, the elderly persons scored higher.

HEALTH

The importance of the health cannot be overlooked in the short discussion on intelligence. This is particularly true in cases of vascular disease, which affect the cerebral cortex and probably influence the brain's capacity to store information. Again, it must be emphasized that each person must be tested as an individual. In addition, it is most important to keep in mind that people who are in an institution are influenced by their surroundings. In many cases, there is no motivation challenge for individuals to test their intellect in a nursing home.

MEMORY AND LEARNING

Memory and learning are functions of the central nervous system. These are slowed down by poor health, bad environment, social intercourse and factors that influence the need for memory and learning. In general, most people see no need to learn new facts, especially if they see no relationship between the old and the new information.

Carl G. Jung, a Swiss psychologist, in his studies of elderly people, saw significant changes in the personality of aged people. Individuals' attention may turn inward in an attempt to find meaning to life. Often he says, individuals will completely change to opposite personalities. He says, "We cannot live the afternoon of life according to the program of life's morning; for what was great in the morning will be little at evening and what in the morning was true will at evening have become a lie" (Jung, 1933).

In relation to the area of change of personality and character, an interesting study was made by Peck (1955). He studied the crucial issues of middle and old age. He sees three issues as central to old age:

1. The individual must establish a wide range of activities so that adjustment to loss of accustomed roles such as those of worker or parent is minimized.
2. Because nearly all elderly individuals suffer physical decline and/or illness, activities in the later years should allow them to stay within the limits of their physical impairment.
3. Although death is inevitable, individuals may in various ways make contributions that extend beyond their own lifetimes; this may provide meaning for life and overcome despair that one's life was meaningless or should have been different than it was.

SEXUAL RELATIONSHIPS

Sexual interests, capacities, and functions change with age. There is a normal decline as part of the aging process. However, this does not mean that older men and women in reasonably good health should not be able to have an active and satisfying sex life. Age and related physiological and anatomical changes are as follows:

1. Older men take longer to achieve full erection and to reach a climax.
2. Tissues lining the vagina are more easily irritated.

3. Uterine contractions become spasmodic and painful.

Chronic physical conditions may affect sexual interest and activity, but his does not have to be total or permanent. Older people need not try to duplicate the sexual behavior of youth in order to enjoy their sexual experiences. Sex is qualitatively different in the later years. It is recreative rather than procreative. Sexual drives and behavior need not necessarily be aimed at achieving orgasm. Most important, sexual activity in the later years may fulfill the human need for the warmth of physical nearness and the intimacy of companionship. Older people should be encouraged to seek this fulfillment.

CHANGES IN SENSORY SYSTEM

Neurosensory changes influence an individual's functioning. Aging affects the individual's ability to function. The world judges people by their responses to everyday stimuli, and in turn, age causes change in these stimuli. In many cases, the elderly person with impaired hearing, vision, or communication may be labeled as stubborn, eccentric, or senile. It is important to know that nerve cells or neurons are lost during the process of aging. With these decreases comes a lessening of the capacity for sending nerve impulses to and from the brain; voluntary motor movements slow down, and the reflex time for skeletal muscles to act is increased. Degenerative changes and diseases involving the sense organs can alter vision, hearing, taste, smell, and touch.

Vision

The aged eye is subject to various changes and disabilities. As a result of the aging process, the retina becomes relatively inflexible, and a tendency toward farsightedness occurs, which leads to the use of reading glasses. The lens of the eye undergoes a yellowing effect. This results in difficulty in discerning certain color intensities, especially blue, green, and violet. The most common diseases of the eye are cataracts and glaucoma. As a result of visual impairment, the older person may suffer serious communication problems. People depend on their vision for receiving and processing a great amount of information about the world. A person's daily living activities involve being able to master various chores that involve sight — sewing on a button, getting dressed in the morning, matching colors for clothes, finding utensils to clean teeth or brush hair are all dependent on vision.

To be able to take care of an elderly person, one must know the amount of vision this person has so he can carry out the tasks assigned to him. Another problem is deciding how much light to allow in the room. If patients have cataracts, they need less light, as it reflects off things and causes a larger degree of vision problems. It is more difficult for people with impaired vision to get around in the dark; thus, if they have to get up in the dark to go to the bathroom, they are apt to fall and hurt themselves. Therefore, a night-light is needed to help people with impaired vision. Some people's vision is impaired by having diminished peripheral vision, especially those who have cataracts. They can see in front of them but often cannot see on the sides.

A person who suddenly has a loss of vision is a frightened person. It is important for the staff to announce themselves when entering this person's presence, letting him know who has entered and why they have come. People who have lost or impaired vision are very self-conscious; they feel slow and awkward and may hesitate to get involved in new activities. Staff should talk to them, always giving them praise for their efforts. They should not be rushed. They need time to develop patience. It might help to put instructions in large letters for these people.

The staff worker in a nursing home should try to understand how it feels to be close to blindness. A good way is for the worker to learn about dimmed vision. He should try tying a handkerchief over his eyes and then try to locate the light switch in a patient's room. Things that could help patients are (1) putting the call switch in a position the patient can reach, and (2) leaving things in the same place in the room so that the patient knows where everything is. If a change must be made, acquaint your patient with the change.

Hearing

The aged person is three times more likely to show a loss of hearing than a younger person. One of the most frequent deficiencies found in the elderly is loss of the ability to perceive higher frequencies. This affects people's speech. They begin unconsciously to slur their words, and this makes them very difficult to understand. It causes speakers to repeat their words many times to shout to the listener. The answer is to speak slowly and in a normal tone of voice. One of the ways of conveying thoughts or feelings that is not used to its fullest is the use of facial expressions. These expressions can convey moods, feelings, excitement, and disapproval.

Many staff workers may not be aware of a patient's hearing loss and after giving them instructions find a limited reaction. This results in an apparent disinterest or evidence of little gratitude for the information they have attempted to deliver. In some cases, the worker goes away, saying that the patient is senile and that is why they cannot communicate with him. It is often very difficult for many of us to put ourselves in the place of the individual who has suffered hearing loss. The Zenith company has produced a record called "Getting Through," which stimulates hearing by its listener and also simulates amplified effects of a hearing aid. It would help a worker to get and listen to this record.

A small hearing test can be carried out by holding a watch to either ear of the patient and moving it away from him by inches at a time. One can soon tell if there is a hearing problem.

Speech or Communications

That which is most common is often neglected until we lose it entirely — speech. Things such as laryngitis, colds, or insensitive tongue due to dental work can impair our speech. In these conditions the effects are temporary; therefore, few give it little mind and care. We rely on accurate information being instantly transmitted to the brain and the brain's ability to respond to these messages.

The human body is complex, and its communication system is one of the most complex of its many systems. Every part of our body assists in receiving, assimilating, and transmitting messages, for example, muscles of the chest supply the power to activate the larynx for producing voice sounds. The structure of the mouth, the nose, and the throat chop the voice up into speech. The eyes and ears pick up important information from all around and the brain coordinates the whole process.

Communication involves getting information about the environment to the brain, processing this information, then transmitting the brain's response back to the environment.

Input (Information to the Brain)

Physical and sensory stimuli attack our bodies from all sides. Each stimulus is converted to neural energy by receptors in the eyes, ears, skin, and tongue. The neural pathways, carrying impulses, go to the brain for appropriate channeling. This results in an act.

Output (Messages from the Brain)

Each step can be eliminated or affected by disease or injury or by psychological causes. One of the most common causes of disruption of comunications is aphasia. Any injury to the brain puts a stop to the line of communication; thus, there is no output. At this time, we know that there are two cerebral hemispheres in the brain, the right and the left. We also know that if a patient has a stroke, the cerebral cortex, say on the left side, is unable to move any part of his body on the right side because the fibers in the cerebral cortex cross over before entering the spinal cord.

Some causes of aphasia are head injuries, broken parts of the brain, cerebral vascular accidents, which cause reduced supply of oxygen to the brain. If the damage is in the dominant hemisphere, left if one is right-handed, aphasia in some degree will be present as well as paralysis of the right side of the body. The reverse is true if the person is left-handed.

It is important to understand what has happened to a patient as a result of his injury in order to be able to help him in his rehabilitation. First, the steps of the communication system must be checked where the failure is:

1. Patient must understand the auditory instructions you have given.
2. Patient must have eyesight to see the written or printed instructions.
3. Patient must be able to differentiate one symbol from another.
4. Patient must label and combine the letters into words in order to

associate them with meaning.

5. Patient must retain the message while keeping it separated from other messages being integrated at that moment.
6. Patient must collect and organize the words into an idea to be spoken.
7. Patient must convert the concept into a series of neural units to be sent down to the motor pathways of the body.
8. Patient must activate the muscles of the speech system in exactly the right sequence to produce the sentences intelligibly.

It is quite obvious that there are many ways that speech can be interrupted.

Testing for Lack of Communication

Visual Reception:
> Do patients wear glasses?
> Can they see out of both eyes?
> Often, if they had a stroke, they cannot see out of one eye. This results in their making adjustments. They will read on one side. If their beds are on the blind side, they are unable to see what is happening on that side. They do not respond the way they should. Check the illumination in the room, check for glare, shadows, and other distracting stimuli that could cause discomfort to the patient.

Visual Perception:
> Determine whether the patient can differentiate basic visual characteristics such as shape, color, and size. Examples of a test would be to place a few objects, such as pictures and letters, in front of him, then hand him one item that is identical with the one of those in front of him, and ask him through speech and gesture to put the item with the one like it in front of him. Repeat with the other items.

Visual Association:
> Have the patient match the printed name with the object or picture or match related items that are similar in structure, such as a knife with a fork, a cigarette with matches, a quarter with a dollar bill.

Touch:

May be affected by peripheral nerve and spinal cord injuries. It could be injuries to the sensory area of the cerebral cortex. The fact that touch, pressure, pain and temperature are impaired can be verified by looking at the chart, because usually the physician will make a note concerning these factors.

Verbal Output or Expression:

If a person gets paralysis due to injury or disease, it will many times affect a patient's speech and expression. The affected side will sag. His tongue will go to the affected side. Another problem with speech is due to poor teeth or dentures that are loose or do not fit.

HOW TO HELP PATIENTS WITH
COMMUNICATIONS PROBLEMS

Staff workers who want to help a patient must first learn all they can about the patient. They must win his confidence, then they must become friends so that when they ask him to do something, he knows they are doing it to help him. After they have succeeded in getting the patient's confidence and he trusts them, they have to learn all about the patient's injury or illness. Now they can start to help the patient in the following ways:

1. Staff should give their thoughts and suggestions in a positive manner to indicate that they know what they are doing.
2. They should be sure to use language that the patient understands.
3. They should look for encouraging signs to praise.
4. If the patient has communication problems, then they must be more patient with him. They must not rush.
5. Staff should try always to carry on the same way all the time, build up a routine.
6. They should look for things that might distract their patient from learning how to do new things.
7. Periodically, they must examine the patient and evaluate him.
8. Another staff worker should make an evaluation for comparison with the first staff member's.
9. The goals staff members are trying to achieve with the patient should be kept in mind while trying to motivate the patient to

achieve these goals.

Staff can achieve their goals if they make the proper approach. In each case, they must judge the patient and then prepare the proper program to rehabilitate the patient to the limit of his ability.

Staff workers of a nursing home must try to get their fellow workers to realize what they are doing for their patient so that if the occasion calls for them to work with the patient, they will not undo all the good that the primary assistants have accomplished. The other workers must be very caring with the patient, who is special to the primary worker. Some suggestions on how to carry out the program are as follows:

1. Do not be in a hurry for fast and dramatic results. This is a long, drawn out affair.
2. Be the same for each session with the patient.
3. Start with an easy job, which the patient can do.
4. Review the previous lesson before going on to new work.
5. Be sure the words used are understandable to your patient.
6. Be sure to relate the material in the lesson to the patient's background.
7. Exhibit humor and friendliness and a relaxed attitude.
8. Watch the patient for signs of fatigue, and as soon as he seems tired, stop.
9. The patient and helper must enjoy the sessions together.

HEALTH CARE

To understand rehabilitation, one must understand health care, for health is what we all seek. The World Health Organization, in their charter defines health as, "The state of complete physical, mental and social well-being and not merely the absence of disease or infirmity."

This concept of health and, later, the definition of rehabilitation are the guides with which we can give proper health care to our patients. We must face the facts that medical care is but one of the many elements contributing to health, even though an improvement in health is seen as a product of medically oriented effort. Success in dealing with problems of health is evaluated largely by such criteria of medical science as disease incidence and life expectancy. Even less precise, and more difficult to measure, are the profound influences of individual living habits, socioeconomic status, attitudes, housing, and education.

AGENCIES FOR HEALTH CARE

Health care in the United States is big business. As a business, it is organized in a variety of ways, each pattern dictated by goals that serve some segment of the health field. No one organization or agency is capable of dealing with all elements of health care. Agencies for health care are classified as (1) government, (2) voluntary, and (3) institutional. There are a great many agencies overlapping each other:

1. Federal Agencies
   a. Department of Health and Human Services, the largest one.
   b. Department of Agriculture, its programs in nutrition and food production contribute to health.
   c. Department of Commerce, it collects censuses and, thus, estimates the needs of the people as related to health.
   d. United States Health Service, its purpose is "Promoting and assuring the highest level of health attainable for every individual and family." Among its functions are —
      (1) to identify health hazards in products and services;
      (2) to support the development of, and to improve the organization and delivery of, comprehensive and coordinated physical and mental health services for all Americans and to provide direct health care services to limited federal beneficiary population, e.g. the indigent, blind, handicapped, and the elderly, etc;
      (3) to conduct and support research in medical and related sciences for further development of health education.
      (4) There are three operating services in Public Health
         (a) Food and Drug Administration
         (b) Health Services and Mental Health Education
         (c) National Institute of Health
2. State Health Organizations
   a. State Department of Health
      (1) Its major aspect is working with local government agencies.
      (2) It also works closely with United States Public Health Services.
3. Voluntary Health Organizations

These contribute to the nation's health programs through —

a. research;
b. direct assistance to patients;
c. public education.

There is a wide variety of primary interest or a specific disease interest; a partial listing of these interests follows.

Alcoholism	Mental health
Allergic disease	Paraplegia
Arthritis	Drug abuse
Birth defects	Genetics
Blindness and sight	Handicapped and crippled
Brain	Hearing
Cancer	Hemophilia
Cerebral Palsy	Multiple Sclerosis
Cystic Fibrosis	Parkinson's disease
Diabetes	Pituitary
Homemaker services	
Kidney	Rehabilitation
Leprosy	Retardation
Lung diseases	Sex education
Medical research	Social disease
	Myasthenia gravis

COMPREHENSIVE CARE

Comprehensive care is a system of personal and family-centered service rendered by a well-balanced, well-organized core of professional, technical, and vocational personnel, who by using facilities and equipment that are physically and functionally related can deliver effective service at a cost that is economically compatible with individual, family, community, and national resources.

PRINCIPLES OF HOMEOSTASIS

Homeostasis is the concept of a comprehensive overview in matters of health. Simply stated, homeostasis is the maintenance of balance of conditions within a system. The concept of homeostasis not only is physiologic but also includes mental and social aspects. Thus, broadly speaking, it includes the following:

1. Body balance; a very fine line
2. Psychological and emotional balances
3. Cultural, social, and political balances
4. Spiritual and philosophic balances

The complexity of health care demands the collaboration of the specialized groups if that care is to have quality and at the same time keep it individual and truly comprehensive.

REFERENCES

1. *Aging and Health: Biologic and Social Perspectives,* by Cary S. Kart, James Metress, and Eileen S. Metress. Addison-Wesley Publishing Co., Menlo Park, California, 1978.
2. *Aging and Behavior,* by Jack Botwinik. Springer Publishing Co., New York, 1973.
3. *Modern Man in Search of a Soul,* C. Jung. Harcourt, Brace and World, New York, 1933.
4. Psychological Development in the Second Half of Life, by R. Peck. *Journal of the American Psychological Association,* 1955.
5. Learning, Motivation and Education of the Aging, by Wilma Donahue. In *Psychological Aspects of Aging,* edited by John E. Anderson. American Psychological Association, Washington, D.C., 1956.
6. A Role Theory Approach to Adjustment in Old Age, by B. Phillips. *Journal of the American Sociology Association,* 1957.
7. *Study of Institutionalized Elderly,* a talk by A. Whanger to the American Gerontological Society, 1975.
8. *The Psychological Aspects of the Aging Process,* by Harold Geist. Warren H. Green, Inc., St. Louis, 1968.
9. Physiological Changes and Diseases, by Ewald W. Busse. In *Care of the Elderly,* edited by A.N. Exton-Smith and J. Grimley Evans. Academic Press in London and Grune & Stratton in New York, 1977.
10. Clinical Manifestation, by A.N. Exton-Smith. In *Care of the Elderly,* edited by A.N. Exton-Smith and J. Grimley Evans. Academic Press in London and Grune & Stratton in New York, 1977.
11. Issues in the Psychiatric Care of the Elderly, by Carl Eisdorfer. In *Care of the Elderly,* edited by A.N. Exton-Smith and J. Grimley Evans. Academic Press in London and Grune & Stratton in New York, 1977.
12. Psychosocial Intervention Programs within the Institutional Setting, by Leonard Gottesman and Elaine Brody. In *Long-Term Care,* edited by Sylvia Sherwood. S.P. Books Division of Spectrum Publishing Inc., New York, 1975.

Chapter 10

ACTIVITIES OF DAILY LIVING

INTRODUCTION

Normal people do many activities without conscious thought. They walk, talk, eat, wash themselves, clean their teeth, and comb their hair. For the handicapped person, however, simple tasks require effort and training. It may be days, weeks, or months before handicapped people can perform to a degree whereby they are independent of care from another individual. It is hard, if not impossible, for normal people to put themselves in the place of the individual who has lost some aspect of his activities of daily living.

The degree to which patients carry out their daily activities determines their independence. In order to determine the activities needed for daily living, we must consider patients' conditions:

1. Are they bedridden?
2. Are they free to move around the nursing home?
3. Are they capable of getting out of the home? If yes, how long?

If a patient is in bed but can do the following, it is felt that they are independent in doing activities of daily living:

1. Feed themselves.
2. Wash themselves.
3. Use the urinal and bedpan.

Yet, they are really not independent because they must depend on others to bring them their food, to bring the materials to wash with, and to bring them the urinals or bedpan.

Let us look at the patients who can move about in the nursing home. These people can go to the bathroom unassisted, they can feed themselves, wash themselves, and dress themselves. Yet, they will need someone to clean the room, make the bed, cook their food, serve it to them, and, in many cases, pick up after them. Patients are not then completely independent if they live in a nursing home. They need some help.

CLASSIFYING PATIENTS

Classifying patients can be done based on levels of care:

1. Nursing Care. If the patient needs help in bathing, feeding, or going to the bathroom or has to have special medications, he needs nursing care.
2. Attendant Care. Someone who needs help with picking up clothes, making the bed, and performing other needs from time to time must have attendants available.

In conclusion, in order to be functional for activities of daily living, one must have ability to (1) be mobile, (2) care for self, and (3) communicate.

LOCOMOTION

The elderly patient who has to lie in bed develops, in many cases, secondary disabilities, both mental and physical, that cause more damage and more problems for rehabilitation than the primary disease. Locomotion has three main objectives:

1. To prevent disease
2. To stimulate and motivate the patient
3. To expand activities of daily living

HOW TO ACHIEVE MOVEMENTS IN BED

The staff of a nursing home must use homemade devices for the specific use for a particular patient's problems. Most elderly patients are accustomed to sleeping in one position, usually flat on their backs or on their sides. In any position they will complain at night that they cannot sleep. Therefore, the staff's first job is trying to move them at least three to five times during the night to new positions. This takes time, yet it has to be done.

To get patients to sit up is a new challenge. One method to do this is to tie a strap or rope to the end of their beds, then they can try to pull themselves up using this method (Fig. 10-1).

Another method to help patients sit up is to have patients use a trapeze and transfer into a chair at the side of the bed (Fig. 10-2).

The use of the side rails has been discussed to aid in movements

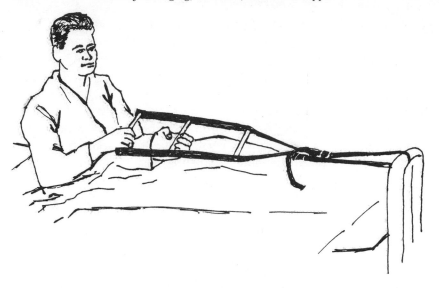

Figure 10-1. Pull-up device. Strap is attached to end of bed, and the other end has a handle to pull up in bed.

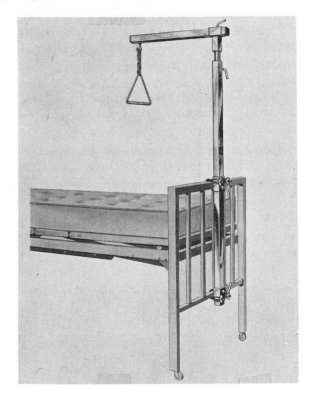

Figure 10-2. Overhead trapeze bar.

of patients.

The type of mattress is very important to a bed patient. It must be firm and hard to enable the patient to move easily and to shift positions. The sheets should be smooth so that the patient can move easily from one position to another. It is important again to emphasize that patients must be taught how to move from bed to chair, from chair to commode, from commode to chair, from chair to bed. These were illustrated by figures in the chapters on hemiplegic patients. Any other patients with weaknesses that do not allow them to move out of bed unless they are urged, helped, and given motivation to do so must learn these movements. An important point to remember in any transfer is that sometimes the patient does not have the strength to move from bed to chair or to commode. A board could then be put across that space to allow a person to slide from one place to another. This has been found useful in some cases. Today manual lifts can help those patients who do not have the strength to move but need to be put into new positions (Figs. 10-3 through 10-6). These manual lifts require one or two attendants, depending upon the weight of the patient. One must be careful if the patient is in such poor condition that he might be hurt or if the patient is quite ill. Also, there is the mechanical hydraulic lift, which can be used to lift patients from a bed to a chair. These are very good and can be bought from any company dealing with rehabilitation products.

WHEELCHAIRS

Wheelchairs are important mobility aids for patients; however, the nursing staff must be careful that patients who could learn to ambulate by themselves do not get into the habit of using a wheelchair and never learn to move about because it is more difficult. Nevertheless, for those patients who are unsteady, uncertain, unsafe, or unfit to try to ambulate, the wheelchair is a marvelous piece of equipment. The standard-size wheelchair can be easily used for all patients with common problems and can be easily adapted to any with special needs. When deciding on a wheelchair, the staff should keep in mind the patient's age, weight, total height standing, and any special aids he might need. Further exploration may be needed when ordering a chair for a patient:

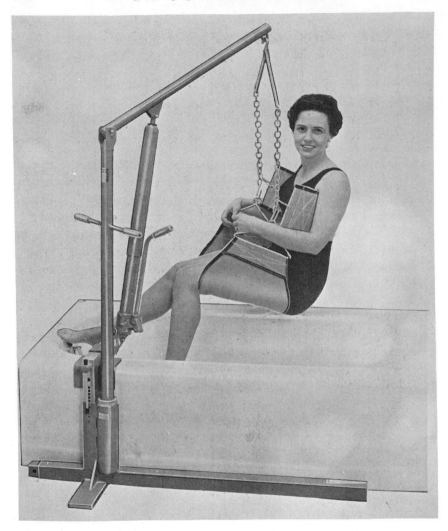

Figure 10-3. Mechanical hydraulic lift for bathtub.

1. Wheelchair with wheels in front. A chair with large wheels in front is more easily propelled by people with impaired shoulder motion and limited elbow motion. However, it is more difficult for an attendant to wheel up curbs or steps. The large front wheels do not permit the chair to be tilted backward as easily as when the large wheels are on the back of the chair.

2. Wheelchair with large wheels in back. The more commonly used

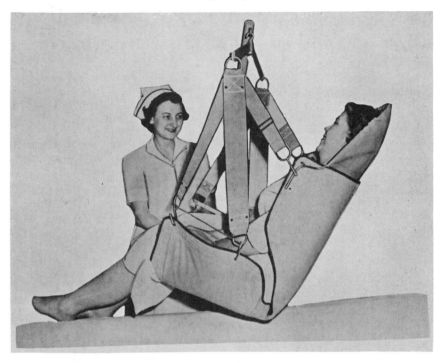

Figure 10-4. Hydraulic lift from bed.

chair is one with 8-inch casters in front. It is more easily maneuvered over rough grounds and curbs.

3. One-arm drive wheelchairs. Chairs that can be propelled with one hand can be purchased by special order.

4. Seat-o-matic® wheelchair. The Seat-o-matic chair has a special seat. A catch can be loosened to a part, allowing it to slide for use of a toilet.

5. Amputee chair. This chair has a special balance to compensate for the loss of weight of an amputated leg.

Other features to be considered in choosing a wheelchair are the following:

1. Small wheels (casters). Eight-inch wheels allow better transportation over rough ground.

2. Caster pins. The use of caster pins to lock casters in place so it is possible to go from front to back in a straight line has advantages.

3. Brakes. Need for brakes is quite obvious; it does not require any

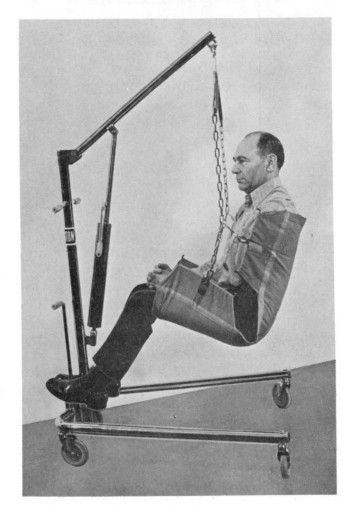

Figure 10-5. Hydraulic lift with casters for movement.

further explanation.

4. Height. The seat should be high enough from the floor to permit full support of the thighs with the feet on the footrests. Also, by sitting further forward in the chair, the feet should rest on the floor.

5. Seat. The width of the seat should be sufficient to accommodate patients' hips comfortably. The depth of the seat should support

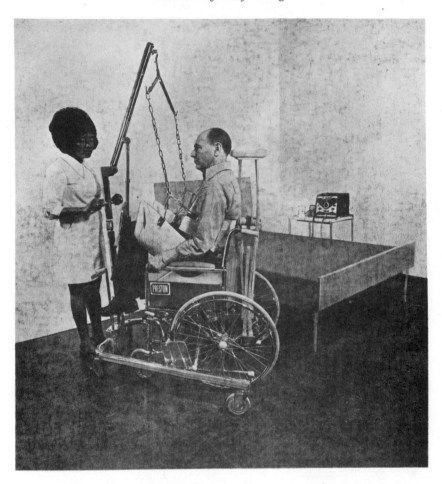

Figure 10-6. Using hydraulic lift from wheelchair.

the thighs to about 2 inches above the knee joint. Some patients put plastic on it so they can slide easily. Some patients put a board under it to make it firm.

6. Backrest. There are different types of backrests. Some recline 45 to 90 degrees, in which case there should also be a headrest.

7. Leg rests. There is the standard leg rest made of metal, which is hinged and can be turned up and out of the way when getting in or out of the chair. Heel straps are used to keep the feet from sliding backwards. Calf straps can swing away, and the entire

footrest swings out. Elevated leg rests can be elevated to any height.

8. Arms. Armrests can be permanent or removeable. They come in wood or can be upholstered.

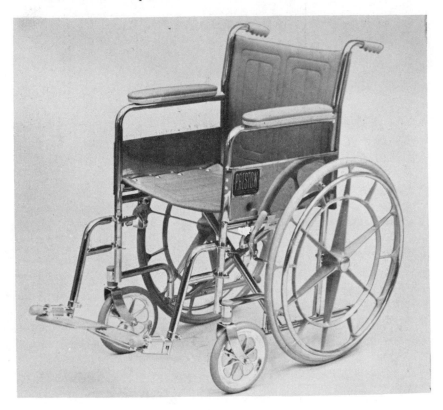

Figure 10-7. Regular wheelchair.

The following body areas must be observed to provide proper sitting and support:

1. Head. Support if patient cannot hold head up.
2. Trunk. Support back if trunk is weak.
3. Forearm. If weakness is in arm or shoulders, provide foream support.
4. Buttocks. Support buttocks but leave knees free.
5. Feet. Feet should be supported.

Maintenance of the wheelchair is important. The wheelchair

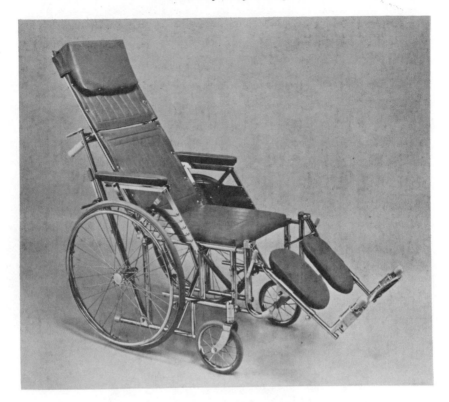

Figure 10-8. Full-reclining wheelchair.

should be cleaned of foreign matter and oiled at least once a week. This will make it last longer and function well for the patient who uses it.

OTHER MEANS OF LOCOMOTION

Locomotion using a cane has already been discussed. Another aid to locomotion is the use of braces. Patients with short leg braces (below the knee), soon learn to ambulate with this aid. Those who have long-legged braces (full length of leg) must learn to put them on and take them off. They must learn how to get in and out of bed and how to get in and out of a chair. Some must learn to use crutches in order to ambulate.

Another type of locomotion is with a walker. The walker is a

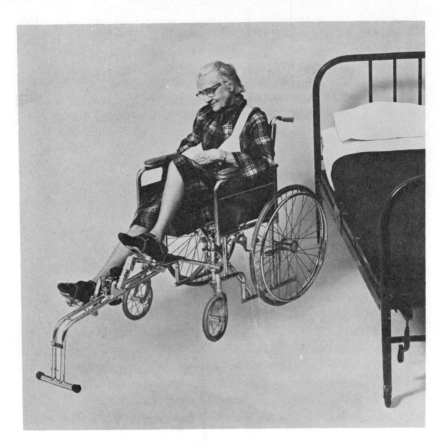

Figure 10-9. Wheelchair with exerciser.

four-legged stand that can be used by a patient by lifting it forward then walking up to it. There are walkers that have casters on them and a seat, which allows the patients to sit down within the walker. They propel themselves forward or backward using their legs for propulsion in the sitting position.

Crutch Walking

Crutches are sticks that are stabilized in at least two places, at hand level and three finger lengths below the axilla, under the arm. There are also Canadian crutches that use two areas of stability, the hand and the forearm.

1. Types of crutches
   a. Regular or underarm crutches
      (1) Adjustable
      (2) Modified for special disabilities
   b. Canadian crutches
      (1) Portion above handhold to midforearm with a half or

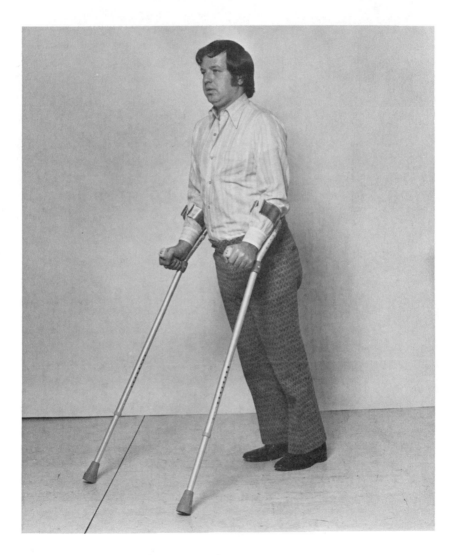

Figure 10-10. Forearm crutches.

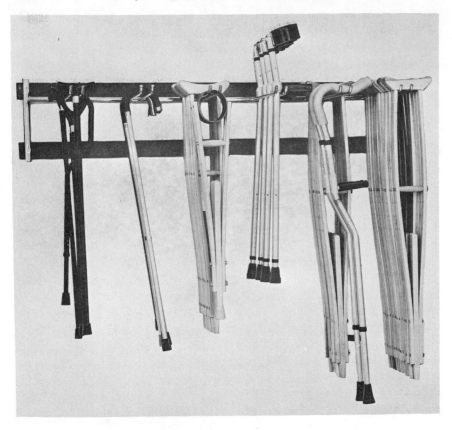

Figure 10-11. Various crutches and canes on a stand.

complete circular leather or metal band attached to
uprights.

  c. Extended canes
    (1) Adjustable and aluminum.
      (a) One upright with extension above handhold at
          125-degree angle to upright. Movable metal partially
          fits around forearm.
  d. Collapsible aluminum crutches.
    (1) Upright has one hinged lock near handhold.
2. Measuring for crutches
  a. Length
    (1) Best method: Patient standing against wall with shoulder
        girdle relaxed and not elevated. Heels should be a few
        inches from the baseboard. Slip a pencil under the arm
        about three finger breadths below anterior axillary

boarder and mark site on wall. Keep shoulders down. Make a pencil mark 6 inches laterally from the heel. Measure distance between marks. This is the total length, including both tips and axillary pads, if used.

(2) Other methods:

    (a) Measure three finger breadths below axilla (shoulder relaxed) to 6 inches out from heel. Allow for heel of shoe.

    (b) Subtract 16 inches from patient's height (this is guesswork because one does not know the length of neck).

    (c) Seventy-seven percent of patient's height.

  b. Height of handholds

This is one of the most important measurements, since the handholds are the fixed points that determine the height the body can be lifted.

(1) Regular or short Canadian crutches

    (a) When holding crutches with wrists hyperextended, the elbows should be flexed at least 30 degrees, keeping the shoulders at normal height.

The importance of correct fitting of crutches in cases of motor disability cannot be overestimated. Frequently, it is a critical factor in whether or not the patient is able to walk with them.

Note: Persons who have never used crutches before will frequently keep the elbows extended and the shoulders elevated. This lessens the load on the triceps. It also makes the crutch look too short. For traumatic cases who are going to be using crutches for a short period of time this is not bad. However, most permanent crutch walkers with uninvolved upper extremities prefer to walk with the elbows flexed.

3. Preparation of crutch walking

  a. Muscle Evaluation

    (1) Strength test

    (2) Coordination

    (3) Contractures

Even if the tests are discouraging, if the patient has the desire to walk, give him a chance. He may be able to accomplish it.

  b. Preparatory exercises

These should be done every hour during the day, stressing the muscles needed for effective use of crutches.

(1) Bed or mat exercises

(2) Wheelchair exercises

(3) Mat exercises with emphasis on walking on hands, and short crutches; also crawling

(4) Standing exercises using horizontal bars or other support to get up

(5) Walking exercises with support other than crutches twice daily

(6) Standing exercises with crutches

Note: Do not allow the patient to fall at this stage or in the early walking. Have several assistants, if necessary, or hold to a belt that has been placed around his waist.

DAILY EXERCISES ON CRUTCHES

1. Walking backward, sideways, and turning around
2. Opening and closing doors
3. Sitting down and arising from a chair
4. Ascending and descending stairs, curbs, and ramps
5. Getting down and up from the floor
6. Falling techniques
7. Clearing obstacles, which is a constant threat
8. Picking up and carrying objects
9. Getting in and out of an automobile, other vehicles

TRIPOD CRUTCH GAIT

The patient maintains a constant tripod position (three points like a tripod).

1. Start both crutches out front and both feet together in back.
2. Move the right crutch.
3. Move the left crutch.
4. Then drag the body and legs forward.

SELF — CARE

Self-care is the term most used in nursing homes. Self-care is the criteria used in placing patients in different areas. It is also the means by which nursing homes decide whether they will take a patient. In the field of rehabilitation, it includes the activities of dressing, bathing, and feeding as the basic issues of activities of daily liv-

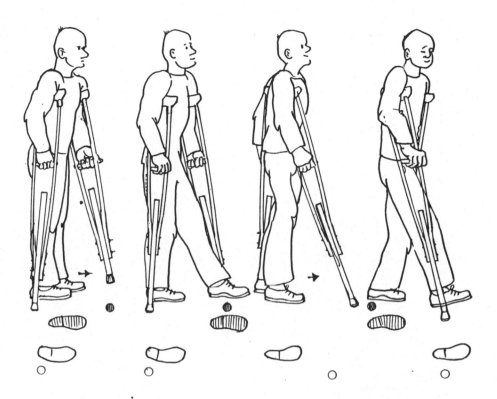

Figure 10-12. Four-point gait. The key to moving in the four-point gait is to move only one crutch or one foot at a time. The illustration shows the following sequence: the left crutch moves, the left foot moves, the right crutch moves, and the right foot moves.

ing. These activities can be divided into the following categories:

EATING. Eating means taking meals in bed and in a wheelchair, using a tray, or in the dining room. The need for special adaptive tools such as special plate or fork or knife or glass may be present if regular equipment cannot be used.

TOILETING. Washing the entire body, either in bed or in a bathtub or shower, combing hair, brushing teeth, using a bedpan or urinal if patient is in bed, using commode if available and can be

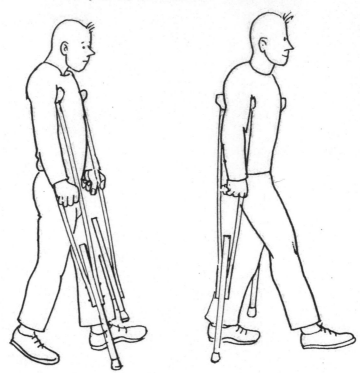

Figure 10-13. Two-point gait. The idea in the two-point gait is to have alternates and opposites move at one time. First the right crutch and left leg move, then the left crutch and right leg move.

used.

DRESSING. Dressing activities includes the use of ordinary or special clothes, changing from day clothes to nightclothes.

MISCELLANEOUS. This category includes smoking, handling of money, opening and closing curtains, using light switches, opening and closing doors and windows, writing, using the telephone, and moving about, whatever the degree or kind.

There are many causes of a disability that can impede a person's doing his own self-care or daily living activities. It is sufficient to say that most patients do lack some ability to do all of their self-care activities. Therefore, we must evaluate the potential of the disabled person to see whether they have any potential for rehabilitation.

Goals for Self-Care

The three steps in making a determination of goals are the following:

1. What self-care activities can or cannot the patient do?
2. As a result of rehabilitation, what might be accomplished?
3. What methods will achieve the goals set for this patient?

It is important to remember that the patient must be considered when making a study of the goals to be achieved. Will they be happy with these goals? Have you discussed the trials and tribulations with the staff and patient as a result of deciding on these goals? Will they make the patient happy during the process of rehabilitation? Sometimes patients are happiest if they are left alone with their disabilities to make their own adjustments to their handicaps, to live out their lives as they wish. One must try to convince the patient of the value of rehabilitation.

Too often rehabilitation professionals make decisions based on their education and experience without considering the most important ingredient, the disabled person. Frequently he has not participated in the planning of these goals. The result in many cases is that goals are not achieved.

There are various methods to achieve self-care, and of course, each disability has specific areas in which the disabled person needs help. There are some general principles that can lay the groundwork for the program for individuals.

PHYSICAL RECONDITIONING. Physical reconditioning includes strength and mobility. Exercises for reconditioning must be based on specific neuromuscular physiology; thus, there are limits to what can be achieved. The staff must be careful not to push beyond the point of achievement; if they do, the patient will become frustrated. It is sufficient to say that staff must strive for the maximal muscle strength possible.

TRAINING PATIENTS TO BE COMPATIBLE WITH THEIR DISABILITIES. For persons to achieve independence, they must be able to cope with their disabilities and work to achieve as much success as possible. To take care of some of their daily living activities, they must achieve some success in their self-care activity program. Most patients are willing to learn if the staff takes the time to teach them. They are willing to learn new techniques to dress, to bathe, or to feed themselves. For example, to teach a hemiplegic patient to put his shirt on by himself, the helper should place a shirt in front of him, tell him to pass his involved arm, with the help of his uninvolved arm, through the sleeve of his shirt, then to lift the shirt up over his head and pass the uninvolved arm into the other sleeve. After two or three tries, he will be able to put his shirt on. This is an achievement of which he can be proud. He can boast about it to the other patients; he can show his family what he has accomplished.

This is only one example of how to teach a patient independence. The same method applies to techniques of feeding. Sometimes the staff must use adaptive and assistive devices to achieve the success for which they are striving. The end result is a patient who can do some of his everyday living activities and the staff workers no longer have to do these things for him. They can go on to other duties that require their time.

ADAPTIVE EQUIPMENT. Another important element in rehabilitation is the use of adaptive equipment and modifications in clothing and in living arrangements. Again, it is worth repeating that there are many companies that have made adaptive devices available for the atypical handicapped person. Some illustrations of adaptive devices are the following: For patients who need help in feeding because they have weak upper extremities and their hands shake, there is a food guard that prevents food from spilling off the sides of their plates. They can push their food up against it in order to pick it up with their utensil (spoon or fork). If the plate moves on the table, they can put a suction cup under the plate, which will keep it immobile. The arthritic patient with a hand problem can use a padded utensil, which allows a better grip for holding a knife, fork, or spoon. Also, if there is limited motion in the shoulder or elbow, there are long-handled or curved tools to allow persons to bring their food to their mouths easier.

In dressing oneself, there are long-handled hairbrushes, long-handled shoehorns, elastic shoelaces, and snaps instead of buttons on shirts, blouses, and bras. Toothbrushes are made in a variety of ways to suit a handicapped person. The toilet might have a higher seat for those too weak to sit down completely. Rails may be mounted by the toilet seat, the bathtub, and the shower for safety or to assist the patient in getting in and out.

People who want to be independent in their self-care activities often get frustrated because they are surrounded by things that are of no help to them. How often does the patient find that the light switch to call the nurse is not available? How often does a person get a telephone call but cannot reach the phone? They wake up during the night and cannot sleep; they want to read but cannot reach the switch to light the bed lamp. The surroundings of the handicapped person must be adapted to their needs.

Some suggestions for arranging a room may be the following: A night table can be placed on each side of the bed, close by for their personal belongings. Their self-care devices should be available for use, for example, the light switches for calling the nurse should be close by and the reading lamp should be where they can reach it. Their adaptive devices should be close so they can use them when they want to and not when the staff worker is around to help them. In short, all of the things that patients need should be placed in a useful position, to be ready when they want to use them. This gives patients the feeling of independence so essential to rehabilitation.

Following is a checklist of self-care activities:

1. Feeding
    a. self
    b. with help
    c. adaptive equipment
    d. use of fork, knife, spoon, cup
2. Ambulation
    a. weight bearing
    b. with help
    c. with cane, crutch, brace, walker
    d. wheelchair
3. Exercise
    a. passive
    b. active
    c. active-resistive
    d. active-assistive
4. Dressing and hygiene
    a. self
    b. with help
    c. adaptive equipment
    d. teeth, shave, etc.
5. Transfer activities

   a. bed to wheelchair
   b. wheelchair to bed
   c. commode
   d. lock wheels
   e. use of chair
6. Bath
   a. self
   b. with help
   c. adaptive equipment
   d. tub, shower, room
7. Positioning
   a. in bed
   b. in wheelchair
   c. in chair
   d. dependent
8. Incidental hand activities (doors, windows, etc.)
   a. self
   b. with help
   c. adaptive equipment

NUTRITION

There is quite a difference of opinion as to the nutritional needs of the elderly handicapped person living in a nursing home. People are individuals with individual problems and needs. The physician in charge will usually discuss the metabolic needs of the patient. The family will tell the staff what a patient ate at home before he entered the nursing home and the types of foods he likes and dislikes. The staff must try to satisfy the physician, the patient, and the family. In some cases, it will be simple, but in most cases it will be a difficult time of adjustment for the patient. Any institutionally prepared food is different from individual cooking. The person who comes from a private home has the biggest adjustment, but those coming from a hospital have to adapt, too.

Patients who come from the hospital may have had an illness; perhaps they could only be fed liquids. Others may have been fed by a tube. It is important to remember that there is no evidence that requirements for nutrients decrease with age. Suggested decreases in food quantity relative to metabolic changes and decreased activity means that the quality of the food must be higher than at an earlier age. In the elderly, as far as caloric needs for everyday living activities, the most significant factor is probably the decreased amount of physical activity. If a person is handicapped, this further reduces his activity.

One of the biggest problems of the handicapped elderly person is obesity. Obesity can complicate other problems such as arthritis, heart disease, and fractures, thus further decreasing physical activities and energy expenditures. This lessened need for calories leaves little room for high caloric foods. Yet, these foods are very popular with the elderly because they are cheaper, easier to chew, and readily available.

In most studies comparing the needs for proteins of elderly people to younger people, there is no substantial difference. There is also no difference or change in the metabolic need for fats as one grows older.

There are some differences in mineral needs; three important minerals that present problems in the elderly are iron, calcium, and potassium. Iron deficiency in the elderly is often caused by poor intake plus an increased incidence of blood loss. Sometimes more meat will help in the absorption of dietary iron. Lack of potassium is very common in the aged patient. It is generally caused by diuretic problems, renal diseases, or diarrhea. The principal source of dietary potassium is in citrus fruits and milk. Yet, these types of foods ar not generally popular with the elderly, and this becomes a problem.

There is no evidence to prove that people need more calcium as they grow older, but normal intake is essential. Also, contrary to some opinions, there is no evidence that people need more vitamins as they grow older. Deficiencies of minerals or vitamins are based on the lack of a balanced diet or on disease, rather than the greater need due to the body aging.

Factor Affecting Nutritional Needs

Nutritional needs can be divided into two categories.
1. Those needs which are the result of metabolic and physiologic changes due to aging.
2. Those needs which affect the amount and types of foods eaten. This includes the social-cultural background of all people, in-

cluding the aged person.

In the first factor, we must point out that as a result of age there is a slowing down of basal metabolism because of a loss of cells and tissue mass and the reduced activity patterns associated with the elderly. Along with these changes, there is a decrease in the capacity of blood vessels to carry nourishment and in the ability of the body to reestablish balances. For example, with a dose of sodium bicarbonate, the body takes eight times longer at the age of seventy years to reestablish the body's sodium level than it would at the age of thirty years. There are other changes in the body's digestive system and absorption capacities as well.

Determinants of Food Intake

To those who have worked with the elderly and those who plan on working with the elderly, it is not necessary to point out that it is important to understand the metabolic and physiologic factors that affect the proper nutrition of aged patients. There are two elements that govern the intake of food:

1. Economics
   Institutions have found that food is one area in which they can economize to meet the demands of making a profit in their businesses.
2. Socializing
   The elderly look on eating as a time for socializing. It is the time when everyone gets out of his room and meets in a shared occasion.

Another element that determines the choices of food that an elderly person eats is physical changes. The loss of teeth or the existence of dentures, with their problems, can lead to a dietary change or modification — foods that are softer and easier to chew. This changes the dietary bulk, which can lead to lower bowel complications. If there are denture problems, it takes the denture wearer four times as long to reach the same level of mastication as a person with his own teeth. This is also true if there are other dental problems. If people do not chew their food properly, they can lose more teeth. The lack of mastication also results in decreased salivary secretions and a tendency toward a dry mouth, which makes chewing and swallowing uncomfortable.

The decreased sense of smell and taste can also influence the patient's food intake. This decrease is due to loss of taste buds of the tongue and receptors in the nose. As a result of decreased taste, people are apt to overseason their food; this in turn can irritate other sensitive parts of the digestive system and in the case of salt contributes to hypertension, heart disease, and kidney malfunction.

Loss of neuromuscular coordination or any neuromuscular disability may lessen food intake also. As people grow older, their coordination declines. Add this to a neuromuscular disorder such as a stroke, Parkinson's disease, or arthritis and there is a complicated problem. These problems lead to inability to handle certain utensils, appliances, or foods. They are often a source of embarrassment, which may interfere with proper nutrition. It often leads to elimination of certain important foods in a person's diet. The psychologic effects of these inabilities and situations have far-reaching consequences to a person's self-image and affect the social function of eating, which is so important at this time in life.

This brings up the topic of special diets, which are difficult to administer in a nursing home and are much more expensive. Also, it singles out some patients, making them different because they cannot eat what others do. This then becomes another psychologic problem.

PSYCHOLOGIC FACTORS. Certain foods cause certain people discomfort. In some cases, this might be on a biophysical basis, and in others its cause is psychological. Certain foods or certain combinations of foods for some people induce symptoms such as heartburn and stomach discomfort. Thus, if patients complain of certain symptoms after they eat, either the combinations of foods should be changed or a physical examination should be given. Of course, if certain foods are to be eliminated, then their nutritional value to the diet must be replaced by another food.

During rehabilitation, the appetite is increased due to renewed physical activity. Exercise is needed to aid in the metabolism of foods and is useful in relieving tension and promoting a sense of physical and mental well-being.

In many cases, income is a primary factor in determining diet in the elderly. Budgeting for food is eliminated when a person goes into a nursing home. However, it must be mentioned that food habits are firmly established in patients before they come to a nursing home, and as such, their diet program has been fixed to a point that they have become accustomed to eating certain types of food. After they enter the nursing home, expense is not their problem. They will be served all kinds of food that they may not have eaten in many years. Trying to change eating habits can make some patients rebel, in which case there is another problem in addition to a physical problem.

Eating is not just a process of providing necessary fuel and chemicals to the human body. It is an important sociopsychologic activity. People eat with people they like. In some cases, the patient who has a special diet uses it to gain friendship of others. It is a social status. Food is important in the expression of religious beliefs, e.g. no meat during Lent and other customs. The elderly use food as a crutch in times of stress and strong emotional disturbances, which occur as a result of an illness or on leaving their home for a nursing home. These emotional stresses cause a loss of appetite and a loss of proteins and calcium balance because of increased excretion associated with stress. Stress can also lead to compulsive nibbling and obesity. Elderly patients who feel rejected or neglected by their family or friends will often use food as an attention-getting device. People may not listen if they say that they are lonely or their leg hurts, but if they are not eating, it worries them, and they begin to pay some attention to patients.

REFERENCES

1. *Self-Help Devices.* Wm. C. Brown Co., Dubuque, Iowa, 1968.
2. J.A. Preston Corporation, 315 Fifth Avenue, New York City, 1978.
3. *Aging and Health,* by Cary S. Kart, James F. Metress, and Eileen S. Metress. Addison-Wesley Publishing Co., Menlo Park, California, 1978.
4. Nutritional Status and Dietary Habits of Older Persons, by E.L. Balcheldor. *Journal of American Dietary Association,* 1957.
5. National Research Council, Recommended Dietary Allowances, Revised 1958.
6. *Manual on Rehabilitation,* edited by Ruby Decker. School of Physical Therapy, University of Texas Medical Branch, Galveston, Texas, 1955.
7. Rehabilitation, Publication No. 713, by Beverly Fahland, on Wheelchair Selection.
8. *Activities of Daily Living,* by E.B. Lawton. Testing and Training Institute of Physical Medicine and Rehabilitation, 1956.

INDEX

R